W9-ANT-093

Nutrient Power

Nutrient Power

William J. Walsh, PhD

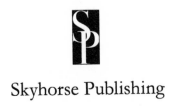

Skyhorse Publishing

Copyright © 2012 by William J. Walsh, PhD

All Rights Reserved. No part of this book may be reproduced in any manner without the express written consent of the publisher, except in the case of brief excerpts in critical reviews or articles. All inquiries should be addressed to Skyhorse Publishing, 307 West 36th Street, 11th Floor, New York, NY 10018.

Skyhorse Publishing books may be purchased in bulk at special discounts for sales promotion, corporate gifts, fund-raising, or educational purposes. Special editions can also be created to specifications. For details, contact the Special Sales Department, Skyhorse Publishing, 307 West 36th Street, 11th Floor, New York, NY 10018 or info@skyhorsepublishing.com.

Skyhorse® and Skyhorse Publishing® are registered trademarks of Skyhorse Publishing, Inc.®, a Delaware corporation.

Visit our website at www.skyhorsepublishing.com

10 9 8 7 6 5 4 3 2 1

Library of Congress Cataloging-in-Publication Data is available on file.

ISBN: 978-1-62087-258-1

Printed in the United States of America

This book is dedicated to my loving mother, Christina, who long ago inspired me with the words "If you can help just one child, all of your work will have been worth it."

Disclaimer

The nutrient therapies described in this book require supervision by an experienced medical professional. Nutrient overloads or deficiencies can have a powerful effect on brain functioning, and improper treatment can cause harm. The brain is a very complex organ, and accurate diagnosis of nutrient imbalances requires testing of blood and urine together with a detailed knowledge of a person's medical history, traits, and symptoms. Readers must not attempt self-treatment based on information in this book.

The case histories in this book provide examples of the treatment approach for specific biochemical imbalances and describe the experiences of real patients. Names and certain other information have been changed to assure patient confidentiality. The case histories are intended to illustrate the clinical process and should not be regarded as evidence of treatment effectiveness.

Finally, *The American Heritage® Dictionary of the English Language** defines mental illness as "Any of various conditions characterized by impairment of an individual's normal cognitive, emotional, or behavioral functioning, and caused by social, psychological, biochemical, genetic, or other factors, such as infection or head trauma." The use of the term mental illness in this book is descriptive only, and no disrespect is intended to the value of the persons experiencing the types of challenges described in this book. The principal objective of this volume is to provide information to help restore health, function, and happiness in the safest way possible.

* *The American Heritage® Dictionary of the English Language,* Fourth Edition, copyright ©2000 by Houghton Mifflin Company. Updated in 2009. Published by Houghton Mifflin Company. All rights reserved.

Acknowledgements

Isaac Newton once said that scientific progress is achieved by "standing on the shoulders of giants." Heroic figures in the field of nutrition include Roger Williams, who established the concept of biochemical individuality; Abram Hoffer, who was the first to demonstrate that nutrient therapy can benefit mental patients; and Carl Pfeiffer, who developed meaningful chemical classifications for schizophrenia. As a young man, I had the privilege of knowing these very dedicated individuals, and I was inspired by their great accomplishments.

My education in the field of mental health started as a volunteer working with ex-convicts released from Illinois prisons. I was surprised to learn that many criminals were raised in good environments along with brothers who had become productive, law-abiding citizens. Several mothers said their offspring who later engaged in criminal activity were clearly different from birth and exhibited shocking behaviors by age two. This led me to a series of experiments at Argonne National Laboratory, where I searched for biochemical abnormalities in violent persons. I am grateful to supervisors Les Burris, Ed Croke, and Walter Massey, who encouraged this work and allowed use of world-class lab facilities. More than a dozen Argonne scientists and engineers generously volunteered their time and talent for the early studies. Our research successes led to the founding of the Health Research Institute in 1982 and the establishment of the nonprofit Pfeiffer Treatment Center in 1989. Jan Olah, Mike Donohue, and Dr. Bob Thomas provided invaluable contributions to this initial clinical adventure. I am forever grateful to the doctors, nurses, and support staff who exhibited great dedication in assisting patients challenged by behavioral disorders, autism, or mental illness. It was a joy working with colleagues who cared more about a patient's welfare than about making money. I am also very appreciative of the volunteer efforts of Ed Tanzman and other board members through the years and to the many donors who provided financial support. Everett "Red" Hodges provided generous research funding during the 1980s. Bruce Jeanes, Judy Nicol, and John Skelton have worked tirelessly in developing our physician training programs along with the indomitable Marion Redstone and her daughter Marnie Lo. Ted DeZurik, Ron Elliott, and Jim Baird provided business expertise that brought financial stability to our charity. Dr. Woody McGinnis was dynamic in developing autism research collaborations. Jeff Tarpey and Aditi Gulabani made important contributions to our research programs. Most of what I've learned about the brain can be credited to Dr. Robert deVito, a psychiatrist and friend who patiently mentored me over the past 12 years.

Financial support for this book was provided by the Hilton Family Foundation based in Panama City, Florida. They were very supportive and patient with me as this 10-month writing project extended past 24 months.

One morning in 1986 at breakfast, Barbara, my wife, asked, "Why don't you quit your job at Argonne today and do what you really want to do?" Her willingness to accept this financial risk while raising five children allowed me to devote the rest of my life to the study of mental illness and development of new medical treatments. Without her constant support and encouragement, my work and this book would not have been possible.

Thanks also go to my outstanding editor, Teri Arranga, for her care in shaping my experiences and thoughts in a way to best serve my vision to help the public. Marlon Irizarry and Tim Rohlwing created the graphics, and Fiona Mayne expertly formatted the manuscript into book form.

Finally, I'd like to express my gratitude to the 30,000 patients whom I've studied over the past 38 years. True understanding of a mental disorder cannot come from laboratory experiments or the scientific literature alone. I found it both educational and inspiring to engage in hand-to-hand combat against mental illnesses in partnership with countless brave patients challenged by these disorders. They have been my greatest teachers.

Contents

Foreword

Psychiatry has made great advances in the past 50 years but needs a new direction. Today's emphasis on prescription psychiatric medications will not stand the test of time. These drugs have helped millions of people diagnosed with depression and other mental disorders, but benefits usually are partial in nature and involve unpleasant side effects. Medication therapy is more art than science, and it involves a considerable amount of trial and error. A fundamental limitation is that psychiatric drugs are foreign molecules that result in an abnormal condition rather than producing normalcy. It is unlikely that psychiatric drugs will ever be universally effective or free of adverse side effects. A new approach is needed. Recent progress in brain science has identified the molecular biology of many mental diseases, and this research provides a roadmap for developing effective drug-free treatments. It is time to move aggressively in this direction.

This book presents a more natural treatment system based on current science that can help millions of persons who have been diagnosed with mental disorders. This approach recognizes that most human beings have nutrient imbalances due to genetic and environmental factors, and these imbalances can cause mischief in many ways, which include the following:

- Serotonin, dopamine, and other key neurotransmitters (chemical messengers that enable brain cells to communicate with each other) are continuously produced in the brain from nutrient raw materials that may be at improper concentrations.

- Nutrient imbalances can alter gene expression of proteins that govern neurotransmitter activity at synapses.

- Deficiency in antioxidant nutrients can cripple the brain's protection against toxic metals.

Neuroscientists have identified the nutrients needed for the synthesis of neurotransmitters, gene regulation, and antioxidant protection, and special blood and urine tests can identify imbalances in these nutrients. Biochemical therapies that use chemicals natural to the body can adjust brain levels of these key nutrients and have a powerful impact on mental health. This approach is more scientific than trial and error use of psychiatric drugs and is aimed at true normalization of the brain. Psychiatric medications have served society well over the past 50 years, but the need for drug therapies will gradually fade away as science advances.

CHAPTER 1

BIOCHEMICAL INDIVIDUALITY AND MENTAL HEALTH

Introduction

History teaches that scientific progress is often blocked not by ignorance but by a widespread belief in something that isn't so. Advances in astronomy were delayed for centuries by assuming that the earth was the center of the universe.[1] Johann Becher's phlogiston theory of combustion[2] was accepted by chemists for nearly a century until Robert Boyle proved it to be false.[3] J. J. Thomson's plum pudding theory[4] of the atom blocked progress in understanding nuclear processes in the early 1900s.

The field of psychiatry has not escaped this malady. The misguided tabula rasa (blank slate) theory championed by English philosopher John Locke in the 17th century[5] persisted as a central belief in psychiatry for 300 years. Locke revived Aristotle's theory[6] that each newborn baby begins life with a "blank slate" with his/her personality and other mental qualities "written" on this slate by life experiences. The blank slate principle was expanded by Freud,[7] Adler,[8] and others who attributed depression, schizophrenia, and other mental disorders to traumatic events, especially those experienced in childhood. This belief led to highly popular psychodynamic therapies that reached their zenith in the 20th century. In 1960, the treatment of choice for mental illness involved a psychiatrist's couch and exploration of negative and positive life experiences. This protocol was dominant in psychiatry for more than 60 years, with benefits reported by millions of patients. However, the approach was very time-consuming and expensive, and progress was frequently partial in nature or nonexistent.

In the 1970s, the tabula rasa theory was proven to be fundamentally wrong, with clear evidence that babies are not born with a blank slate but rather with strong predispositions that affect personality and behavior. This understanding has led to a revolution in mental health, with a new focus on the biochemistry of the brain.

The Biochemical Revolution

Psychiatry research from 1950-1970 included several well-designed studies that examined the impact of life experiences on depression, bipolar disorder, schizophrenia,

1

and other mental illnesses. The studies confirmed that a history of emotional or physical trauma, poverty, and deprived living conditions increased the likelihood of these disorders. However, this effort produced a surprising result—the discovery that the greatest predictor of mental illness was not life experiences but rather a family history of the same disorder. The most decisive results came from adoption and twin studies[9-11] that confirmed the presence of powerful predispositions that could not be explained by tabula rasa. By the mid-1970s, most scientific and medical experts agreed that the dominant cause of most mental illness involved genetic or acquired chemical imbalances that alter brain functioning. Within a few years, psychiatry researchers changed their focus from life experiences to neurotransmitters, receptors, and the molecular biology of the brain.

It soon became apparent that brain chemistry is extremely complex and that clear understanding of the neurobiology of mental illness would require decades of research. With millions of mentally ill persons needing immediate treatment, the psychiatry profession turned to the only known method of altering brain chemistry—psychiatric medications.[12] From the beginning, there were many seriously ill persons who benefited from these medications. Unfortunately, the improvements usually were partial in nature and resulted in serious side effects. Early medications included Prolixin, Mellaril, Haldol, and Thorazine, which frequently resulted in sedation, personality change, weight gain, loss of libido, and other nasty symptoms. Over the past 30 years, many improved medications have been developed, including selective serotonin reuptake inhibitor (SSRI) antidepressants and atypical antipsychotics. However, serious side effects continue to be reported for each of these newer medications, and there is little hope that future psychiatric drugs will ever be free of this problem.

It seems likely that advanced treatments in future years will utilize natural body/brain chemicals that restore the patient to a normal condition rather than foreign drug molecules that result in an abnormal condition. The acceleration in scientific knowledge regarding neurotransmitters, receptors, and the molecular biology of the brain is greatly assisting achievement of this goal. The world will eventually learn the wisdom of Pfeiffer's Law: "For every drug that benefits a patient, there are natural substances that can achieve the same effect."

The Birth of Neurotransmitters

The human brain is an organ of extraordinary complexity.[13-14] A typical adult has approximately 100 billion brain cells, with an average of 1,000 synaptic connections per cell. Every thought, action, and emotion involves communications between

It is now clear that abnormal levels of key nutrients can have an adverse effect on brain chemistry and mental health. Because of these abnormalities, some individuals have a predisposition for conditions such as clinical depression, oppositional defiant disorder (ODD), and attention-deficit/hyperactivity disorder (ADHD), while others are quite invulnerable to these disorders. Biochemistry can be affected by diet and stressful life events, but the dominant factor often goes back to genetics or, additionally, epigenetics. The concept of epigenetics will be addressed more thoroughly in Chapter 4, but very briefly, the environment (e.g., diet, toxins, lifestyle) can affect the expression of a person's genes, and this alteration in gene *expression* is called epigenetics. Epigenetics explains why one identical twin may manifest a particular disease, while the other does not.

A comprehensive metabolic analysis of any person would likely reveal several nutrients that are deficient due to genetics. Some deficiencies might be of minor importance with respect to human functioning, while others could result in serious mental problems. If people knew which nutrients were deficient, they might benefit greatly from many times the recommended daily allowance (RDA) of those nutrients since they may be fighting a genetic tendency for deficiency.

After clinical experience with thousands of mental health patients, I was surprised to learn that nutrient *overloads* usually cause more mischief than deficiencies. This explains why most multivitamin/mineral products are ineffective for mentally ill patients and can cause more harm than good. Patients with an overload of copper, methionine, folic acid, or iron are likely to deteriorate if they take supplements containing these nutrients. In most cases, mentally ill persons cannot become well using a special diet or indiscriminately stuffing themselves with amino acids, vitamins, and minerals.

The challenge is to carefully identify the specific nutrient overloads and deficiencies possessed by an individual and to provide treatments that normalize blood and brain levels of these chemicals with rifle-shot precision. This is the essence of biochemical therapy.

CHAPTER 2

BRAIN CHEMISTRY 101

The Chemical Symphony of the Brain

Every perception, thought, emotion, action, and memory involves a complex symphony of chemical processes in the brain. The sciences of neuroanatomy and neurochemistry have achieved great progress in the past 200 years, resulting in a basic understanding of the structure of individual, tiny brain cells and the chemical events that dominate brain function.

Brain cells were discovered in the early 1800s by Jan Evangelista Purkinje,[17] Carmillo Golgi,[18] and others using high-magnification microscopes and tissue staining methods. For several years, it was believed that brain cells (called neurons) were directly wired together forming a complex electrical circuit. However in the 1880s, Spanish scientist Ramon y Cajal[19] discovered that neurons didn't actually touch but communicated by sending signals to nearby neurons. At first, the signals were described as sparks that jumped from neuron to neuron. In the 1890s, Charles Sherrington's laboratory[20] in England developed convincing evidence that the transmission was chemical in nature and occurred across a tiny gap between brain cells that he called a synapse from the Greek word meaning "to clasp."

In 1921, Austrian scientist Otto Loewi discovered the first neurotransmitter, which is now known as acetylcholine.[21] Many dozens of neurotransmitters have been identified among the more than 100 in the human brain. Much research has been devoted to neurotransmitters that are associated with specific mental disorders including depression (serotonin), schizophrenia (dopamine, glutamate, serotonin), anxiety (norepinephrine, GABA), and Parkinson's disease (dopamine).

Neurons are cells that receive, process, and transmit electrochemical signals at a speed of about 200 mph. In addition to the approximately 100 billion neurons in the brain, glial cells[22] provide structural support and nourishment for the neurons and are far more numerous than neurons. Most neurons vary in size from 4 microns to 100 microns in diameter. Their length varies from a fraction of an inch to several inches. As shown in Figure 2-1, neurons consist of a cell body with branching dendrites (signal receivers) and a long, wire-like projection called an axon, which conducts the nerve signal. The axon terminals transmit the electrochemical signal across a synapse (the gap between the axon terminal and the receiving cell).

The neuron's nucleus contains the individual's DNA, which is neatly wrapped around tiny proteins called histones. A typical neuron has 1,000 hair-like dendrites branching from the cell body with a receptor at each terminal that can receive chemical messages from nearby brain cells. A typical human brain has approximately

Figure 2-1. Neuron

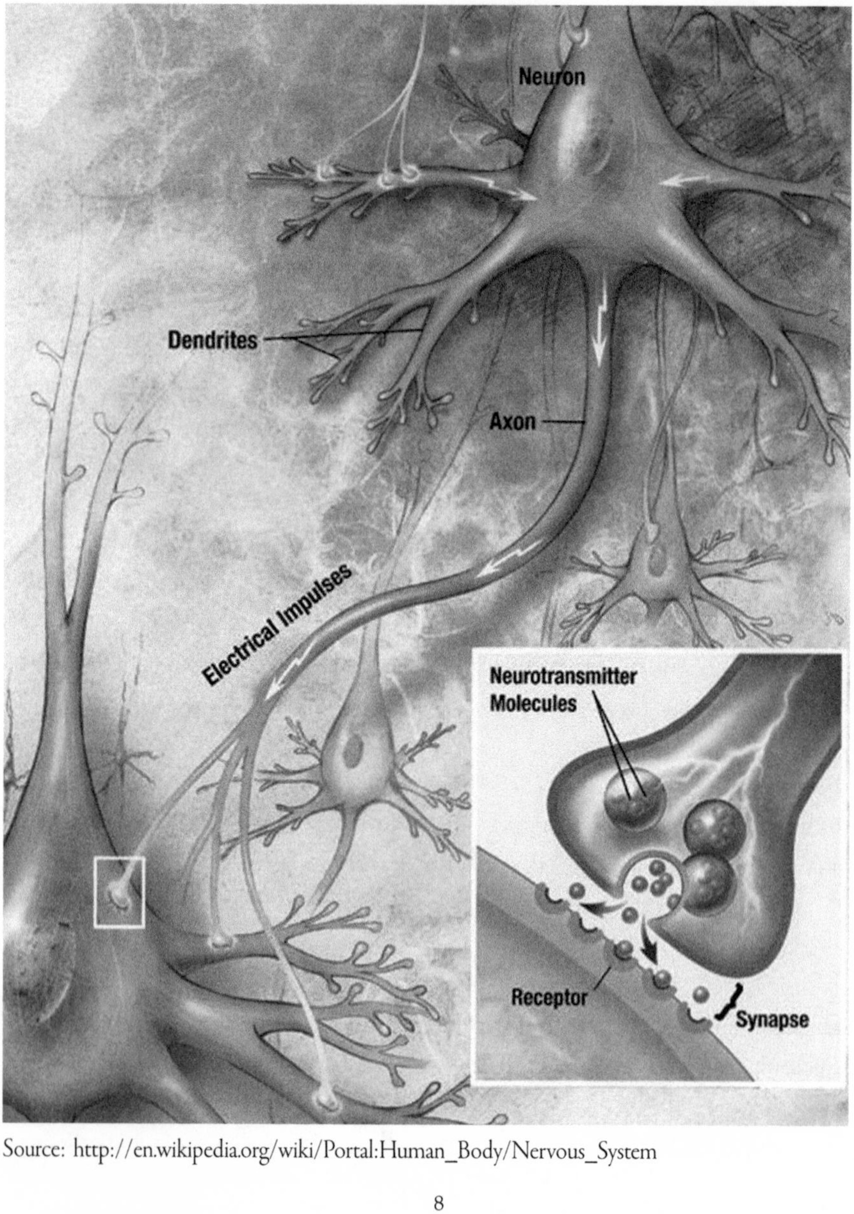

Source: http://en.wikipedia.org/wiki/Portal:Human_Body/Nervous_System

100 trillion receptors. The axon is coated and insulated by a substance called myelin, which consists of 70-80% lipids (fat) and 20-30% protein.

Brain neurons act as tiny battery cells that are free-floating; in other words, in most cases, they do not actually touch other neurons. They typically develop a resting voltage of about 1/15 volt from ion concentration gradients across the membrane. When activated, the neuron acts as a miniature gun that shoots neurotransmitter molecules into a synapse. Like snowflakes, no two neurons are exactly alike. They differ in shape and the voltage threshold needed to fire. A neuron will switch on only if its resting threshold voltage is exceeded. Each neuron receives a multiplicity of inputs from its dendrite receptors, some that promote cell firing and others that are inhibitory. When a neuron fires, an electrochemical pulse called an *action potential* is sent down the axon to the terminus, releasing neurotransmitter molecules into the synaptic space. Some of these molecules link with receptors of nearby cells, sending an activating signal to that cell. This is the basic way in which brain cells communicate with each other. If a sufficient number of brain cells are activated, a thought or action can result.

A neuron that sends a signal across a synapse is called presynaptic, and the neuron that receives the signal is termed postsynaptic. The receptors themselves may be thought of as hunks of protein embedded in the membranes of neurons. Most receptors have a unique configuration that can receive a signal from only one type of neurotransmitter. In general, a serotonin receptor can be activated by serotonin molecules alone and not by other brain chemicals.

The Neurotransmitter Life Cycle

Most neurotransmitters are produced by chemical reactions in brain cells. After a period of service, they are chemically degraded. The life cycle steps are as follows:

1. Synthesis (generation by chemical reaction)
2. Packaging into vesicles
3. Release into a synapse
4. Interaction with an adjacent cell
5. Reuptake (transport back to the original cell for reuse)
6. Death (deactivation by chemical reaction)

Step 1: Synthesis: Most neurotransmitters are produced in the axon terminus near the synapse. The reactants consist of (a) amino acids and other nutrients that enter the cell through the cell membrane, and (b) enzymes that are produced by gene expression in the nucleus and make the long journey down the axon via microtubule tunnels.

Step 2: Packaging into vesicles: Vesicles[23] are storage units that resemble tiny bubbles swimming in the cell liquid (cytosol). They are also formed in the nucleus and travel down the axon via microtubule tunnels. Neurotransmitters are loaded into vesicles through proteins called vesicular monoamine tranporters (VMAT)[24] that are embedded in vesicle membranes. About 20 to 200 neurotransmitter molecules can be stored within each vesicle. Some of the vesicles attach to the neuron's membrane at docking sites where they can launch their neurotransmitters into the synapse.

Step 3: Release into a synapse: When a brain cell fires, calcium ions (Ca^{++}) rush into the cell, causing vesicles to be ripped open and neurotransmitter molecules sprayed into the synapse. The ruptured vesicles are either absorbed into the cell membrane or returned to the cytosol liquid for formation of new vesicles.

Step 4: Interaction with an adjacent cell: A fraction of the neurotransmitter molecules travel across the synapse to receptors of nearby cells and transmit a chemical message that either promotes or inhibits cell firing. For example, glutamate neurotransmitters are excitatory and tend to promote cell firing. In contrast, GABA neurotransmitters are usually calming and inhibit cell firing. After a brief interaction, the neurotransmitter molecule is released from the receptor back into the synapse.

Step 5: Reuptake: Neurotransmitter molecules can be quickly returned to the original cell through transmembrane transporter proteins and packaged into new vesicles for reuse. This reuptake process usually dominates neurotransmitter activity at synapses, and transporters are the target of most psychiatric medications. For example, SSRI antidepressants directly interact with transporters to inhibit serotonin reuptake and increase serotonin concentrations in the synapse.

Step 6: Death: Neurotransmitter molecules eventually undergo chemical degradation that removes them from the scene. For example, monamine oxidase reacts with a fraction of serotonin molecules in the synapse. In addition, some neurotransmitter molecules diffuse away from the synapse and are lost by that mechanism. Figure 2-2 shows the synapse between a brain cell and a dendrite receptor of a neighboring brain cell.

Most psychiatric medications[12] work by altering neurotransmitter activity at synapses. As described previously, SSRIs disable transporters, thus slowing the exit of serotonin from the synapse. The serotonin molecules are essentially trapped in

Figure 2-2. Schematic of a Brain Synapse

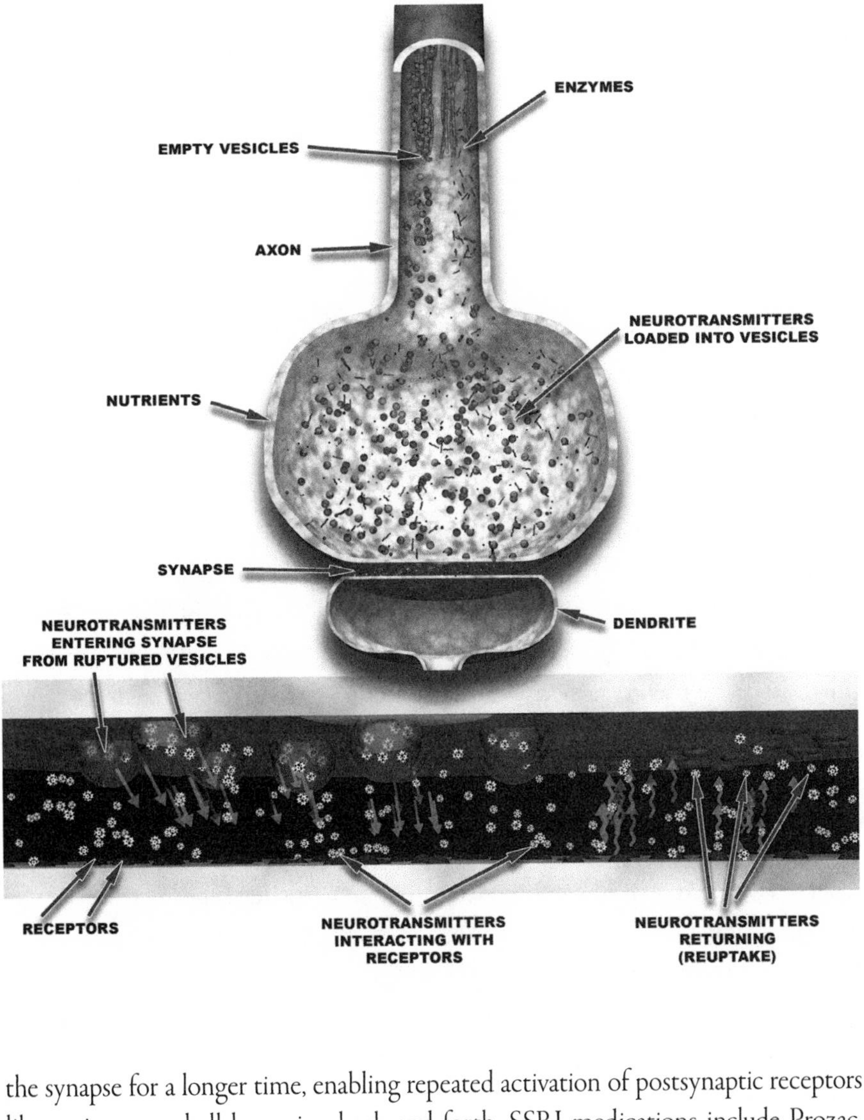

the synapse for a longer time, enabling repeated activation of postsynaptic receptors like a ping-pong ball bouncing back and forth. SSRI medications include Prozac, Zoloft, Paxil, Luvox, Celexa, and Lexapro. Effexor, Cymbalta, and Pristiq are selective serotonin and norepinephrine inhibitors (SNRIs) that increase synaptic activity of both serotonin and norepinephrine. Another class of antidepressants are the monoamine oxidase inhibitors (MAOIs), which reduce levels of monoamine oxidase, a natural biochemical that destroys a fraction of the serotonin molecules in the synapse. MAOI drugs often involve serious side effects and have generally been replaced by SSRIs.

Benefits of biochemical therapy

An alternative treatment approach is offered by biochemical therapy, which represents a natural method of correcting imbalances in neurotransmitter activity. The clinical challenge is to determine the biochemistry of each patient and to develop an individualized treatment aimed at normalizing brain chemistry. This medical modality should be supervised by a licensed practitioner experienced in therapeutic use of vitamins, minerals, amino acids, and essential oils. For most patients, the benefits of biochemical therapy result from the following:

- Normalizing the concentration of nutrients needed for neurotransmitter synthesis
- Epigenetic regulation of neurotransmitter activity using targeted nutrient therapy
- Reducing free-radical oxidative stress

For example, many patients suffering from depression exhibit low levels of vitamin B-6, an important cofactor in the last chemical step in serotonin synthesis. These patients may benefit from Prozac or another SSRI medication, but nutrient therapy that normalizes brain levels of B-6 may be equally effective. In another example, methylating nutrients such as S-adenosylmethionine (SAMe) can inhibit gene expression of serotonin transporters and, therefore, increase serotonin activity. For many patients, antioxidant nutrients can assist in normalizing activity at GABA, N-methyl-D-aspartate (NMDA), and other receptors.

A major advantage of biochemical therapy is the absence of the serious side effects associated with psychiatric medications. This medical approach uses natural chemicals rather than molecules that are foreign to the brain and induce an abnormal condition. Biochemical therapy can be used together with medication and counseling, providing great flexibility to the mental health practitioner. As brain science advances, biochemical therapy may gradually replace psychiatric drugs as the treatment of choice for mental illnesses.

CHAPTER 3

THE DECISIVE ROLE OF NUTRIENTS IN MENTAL HEALTH

The Brain – A Chemical Factory

Considering the complexity of brain chemistry and the multiplicity of gene processes that could go wrong, it is surprising that more humans do not have serious mental problems. Effective brain function requires a proper concentration of neurotransmitters in specific areas of the brain. These complex chemicals are continuously produced by enzymatic reactions within special brain cells. For example most of our brain's serotonin is synthesized in the *raphe nuclei* along the brainstem and transported by axons to areas throughout the brain. In another example, dopamine is produced in several areas of the brain, including the *substantia nigra* and the *ventral tegmental area*.

As mentioned in Chapter 1, the primary raw materials for neurotransmitter synthesis in the brain are nutrients: amino acids, vitamins, minerals, and other natural biochemicals. The levels of these ingredients are well-regulated for most persons, but gene abnormalities can result in a nutrient deficiency or overload. The net result can be an abnormal neurotransmitter concentration and a serious mental illness. Psychiatric medications can be effective in coping with neurotransmitter imbalances. However, as we have emphasized, advanced nutrient therapy to promote normalization of neurotransmitter levels in the brain can also be effective, with the advantage of reduced adverse side effects.

Database Studies, Early Nutrient Therapies, and Beyond: Examples from Schizophrenia

Canadian psychiatrist Abram Hoffer[25] was an early pioneer in nutrient therapy for schizophrenic patients. In 1951, Hoffer and his colleague Humphrey Osmond began experimenting with high doses of niacin and reported major reductions in auditory hallucinations and other schizophrenia symptoms. They conducted six double-blind, placebo-controlled experiments that yielded impressive evidence of improvement in the niacin group. Best results were reported for young schizophrenics, with lesser efficacy for chronic patients. After many years of research, Hoffer recommended a protocol involving the combined use of niacin, folic acid, vitamin B-12, vitamin C, essential oils, and special diets for schizophrenic patients.

Dr. Hoffer theorized that schizophrenia resulted from excessive levels of adrenaline and adenochrome (breakdown products of dopamine and norepinephrine), and his therapy was aimed at normalizing brain levels of these chemicals. However, new epigenetics research indicates that folates and niacin can powerfully reduce dopamine activity by enhancing acetylation of histones (see Chapter 4). This mechanism may be responsible for the thousands of reports of benefits from Hoffer's protocols. In collaboration with Dr. Carl Pfeiffer, Hoffer's group also discovered a condition termed *pyroluria* or the *mauve factor* that is the dominant imbalance in about 20% of schizophrenics. They identified pyroluria as an inborn disorder resulting in severe deficiencies of zinc and vitamin B-6. Hoffer's therapy approach became known throughout the world and was used by hundreds of doctors over the next 20 years. In 1973, an American Psychiatric Association (APA) task force reviewed a large number of published, controlled studies and concluded that Hoffer's claims of efficacy were not justified.[26] This finding was very controversial and continues to be debated today. Hoffer's nutrient therapy has never been accepted by mainstream medicine, but doctors throughout the world continue to use his methods. This modality is still championed by the International Society of Orthomolecular Medicine and the *Journal of Orthomolecular Medicine.*

The possible role of pyrroles in mental health was identified more than 50 years ago when researchers noticed that urine samples of certain psychotic subjects developed a reddish-purple or mauve color. When these individuals were found to possess similar traits and symptoms, the mauve factor became a subject of active research. Hoffer and Pfeiffer reported that more than 20% of schizophrenics exhibited mauve urine. In collaboration, their research groups isolated the mauve chemical and found it to be a pyrrole. For many years, this chemical was misidentified as kryptopyrrole and the medical condition termed pyroluria. The actual source of the mauve coloration is the complex chemical hydroxyhemopyrrolin-2-one (HPL). The syndrome of elevated pyrroles is now termed *pyrrole disorder* or *mauve.* In 2006, McGinnis and colleagues published an extensive review of pyrrole chemistry and its role in mental health.[27]

Hoffer's early work inspired a prominent American doctor, Carl Pfeiffer, MD, PhD, to study the role of nutrients in mental illness. While working at a research hospital in the late 1950s, he discovered abnormal blood chemistry in a catatonic patient who had been nearly motionless for months. Pfeiffer treated the man with an intravenous cocktail of amino acids, vitamins, and minerals, and within seven days, the man experienced a near-complete recovery. The hospital instituted a study to determine the reason for his sudden ability to walk, talk, and behave normally but concluded that Pfeiffer's nutrient therapy had no role in his improvement. The patient voluntarily stopped Pfeiffer's nutrients and within two weeks returned to his catatonic state. Pfeiffer then cycled the man in and out of his catatonia several times, but his medical director refused to believe that nutrients were responsible. This was the beginning of Pfeiffer's difficulties with mainstream medicine, and it launched him on a new career researching the use of nutrient therapies for mental illness. Pfeiffer eventually concentrated his efforts on schizophrenia and founded the Princeton Brain Bio Center in Skillman, New Jersey.

Pfeiffer evaluated more than 20,000 schizophrenics and developed the world's largest chemistry database for this condition. His greatest contribution was the discovery of individual schizophrenia biochemical types, each with distinctive symptoms and blood/urine chemistries.[28-29] This finding was in harmony with the widespread belief that schizophrenia is an umbrella term that includes several different mental disorders. Pfeiffer identified body chemistries and symptoms and recommended individualized nutrient therapies for each biotype. He reported that 90% of schizophrenics fit into one of the three major biochemical types that he called histapenia, histadelia, and pyroluria, with an additional 4% suffering from wheat gluten allergy. He also identified several low-incidence disorders that could cause schizophrenia symptoms, including porphyria, homocysteinuria, hypothyroidism, and polydipsia.

Pfeiffer believed that histamine deficiency (histapenia) and copper overload were responsible for classic paranoid schizophrenia that usually involved auditory hallucinations. He treated this condition with folic acid, vitamin B-12, niacin, zinc, and augmenting nutrients. In contrast, Pfeiffer's histadelia (histamine overload) biotype typically involved delusions or catatonic behaviors that he treated with methionine, calcium, and sometimes with antihistamines. Another 20% of schizophrenia patients fit into Pfeiffer's pyroluria biotype that was often characterized by both auditory hallucinations and delusions. Pfeiffer treated the pyrolurics with strong doses of vitamin B-6 and zinc.

Histamine is a neurotransmitter, and Pfeiffer believed that abnormal histamine levels were the underlying cause of most cases of schizophrenia. His treatments concentrated on normalizing histamine levels in the brain. In the early 1990s, I amassed evidence that methyl and folate levels had a far greater impact on mental health than histamine and concluded that histamine was not a decisive factor in schizophrenia. For example, hundreds of patients achieved impressive recoveries while their abnormal histamine levels remained unchanged. It appears that Pfeiffer developed effective nutrient therapies but proposed the wrong theory to explain their efficacy. Today, blood histamine is used as a marker for methylation status but not for mental status. Histamine and methyl groups are present in measurable levels throughout the body and an inverse relationship exists between them. Eventually, Pfeiffer's terms histadelia and histapenia were replaced by *undermethylation* and *overmethylation*, with the understanding that serotonin, dopamine, and norepinephrine activities are powerfully influenced by methyl status. However, this approach did not explain why a powerful methylating treatment (folic acid and vitamin B-12) caused dramatic worsening in undermethylated schizophrenics. This problem was resolved in 2009 with the discovery that methyl and folate have opposite epigenetic impacts on neurotransmitter reuptake at synapses.

The activities of serotonin, dopamine, and norepinephrine neurotransmitters in the brain are dominated by transporters present in the membranes of presynaptic brain cells. You may recall from our earlier discussion that the transporters enable the return of neurotransmitters to cells after they are sprayed into a synapse. This process is called reuptake, and most modern psychiatric drugs are aimed at altering transporter function. The genetic expression of transporters is inhibited by methylation and enhanced by acetylation, processes which are described in Chapter 4. Acetylation is the process of adding an acetyl group (CH_3CO) to a molecule. The relative amounts of methyl and acetyl attached to DNA and histone tails impact the synaptic concentration of reuptake proteins and the activity of dopamine, serotonin, and norepinephrine. By different mechanisms, folates and niacin promote dominance of acetylation at DNA and histones (see Chapter 4). Methionine and SAMe produce the opposite effect by promoting methylation of DNA and histones. The net result is that activities of serotonin, dopamine, and other neurotransmitters are strongly influenced by the methyl/folate ratio. After 25 years of searching, we finally have a convincing explanation for the apparent effectiveness of folate, niacin, and methylation therapies developed by Abram Hoffer and Carl Pfeiffer.

Dr. Pfeiffer[28-29] and I[30] studied more than 30,000 patients with a diagnosis of mental illness and an additional 15,000 with a behavioral disorder (BD), ADHD, or autism. These evaluations have generated millions of laboratory analyses measuring the concentrations of biochemical factors in blood, urine, and tissues. Comparison with known normal levels for healthy persons reveals a very high incidence of chemical imbalances in these clinical populations. Considering the vast amounts of data, it is extremely unlikely that this is a coincidence.

Thousands of Pfeiffer's schizophrenic patients reported improvement, but the absence of published controlled studies measuring treatment effectiveness of Pfeiffer's nutrient protocols prevented acceptance of his protocols by mainstream medicine. Prior to his death in 1988, Pfeiffer was nominated for a Nobel Prize (which he didn't win) and was widely regarded as the world's leading expert in biochemical therapy. Pfeiffer's nonprofit Princeton Brain Bio Center experienced financial problems in the 1990s and no longer exists.

The work of Carl Pfeiffer has been continued by several doctors and clinics in the two decades since his death. Dr. Pfeiffer trained numerous physicians in his protocols, and these therapies are still used by complementary medicine practitioners throughout the world.

I had the privilege of collaborating with Pfeiffer in the evaluation of 500 patients diagnosed with behavioral disorders or mental illness over a 12-year period. After a few years of prodding by Dr. Pfeiffer, I founded the nonprofit Pfeiffer Treatment Center in Illinois, which treated more than 25,000 patients, including thousands diagnosed with schizophrenia. In the early years, the Pfeiffer Treatment Center treatment methods duplicated the lab testing, medical history, diagnosis, and treatment protocols of the Princeton Brain Bio Center. In subsequent years, we introduced improvements as brain science progressed and the impact of key nutrients on neurotransmitter activity became clearer. In 2008, I left the Pfeiffer Treatment Center to develop an international physician training program. Sadly, the Pfeiffer Treatment Center experienced financial problems and closed its doors in July 2011. Fortunately, there are many talented physicians throughout the world who are now quite expert in these treatment protocols.

Coping with Biochemical Imbalances

Longitudinal studies over the past 30 years indicate that a person's biochemical tendencies persist throughout life, suggesting that these tendencies are genetic or epigenetic in origin. In many cases, symptoms of a particular imbalance have been clearly evident since age two, for example, as in the case of cruelty to childhood pets. The impact on a person's life depends on the severity of the chemical imbalance and on exposure to environmental factors. For example, a child with a mild tendency for aggressive behavior may develop normally if there is a good diet, an absence of serious traumatic events, and a nurturing family. However, a child born with the severe chemistry observed in serial killers (see Chapter 8) is likely to become a criminal unless brain chemistry is corrected. Counseling and a good environment may be effective in mild-to-moderate behavioral disorders, but a severe chemical imbalance cannot be loved away, and treatment must focus on correcting brain chemistry. Similarly, a mild genetic tendency for depression may be overcome by factors such as a good environment, exercise, and counseling, whereas a severe tendency may require aggressive biochemical intervention. All of these patients are good candidates for individualized nutrient therapy.

The Repeat Offenders

For several years I was perplexed by the repeated presence of certain biochemical imbalances in completely different mental disorders. For example, copper overload is present in most cases of hyperactivity, learning disability, postpartum depression, autism, and paranoid schizophrenia. In another example, undermethylation is often present in antisocial personality disorder, clinical depression, anorexia, obsessive-compulsive disorder, and schizoaffective disorder. The primary repeat offenders are the following:

+ Copper overload
+ Vitamin B-6 deficiency
+ Zinc deficiency
+ Methyl/folate imbalances
+ Oxidative stress overload
+ Amino acid imbalances

Eventually, I realized these factors had something in common—a direct role in the synthesis or functioning of a major neurotransmitter. It seems most unlikely that this is a coincidence. The situation is complicated since a mental illness may involve more than one imbalance. For example, antisocial personality disorder associated with criminality usually involves the combination of zinc deficiency, oxidative overload, undermethylation, and elevated toxic metals. Paranoid schizophrenia usually involves overmethylation, folate deficiency, and elevated blood copper. Because of genetic variations, a particular chemical imbalance may have a variety of outcomes for different persons. Each of these offending chemical imbalances can be effectively treated without the use of psychiatric medications.

Remediating the Repeat Offenders

Copper overload

In the early 1800s, W. Meissner[31] identified the presence of copper in all forms of life. We now know that copper plays an important role in the synthesis of neurotransmitters,[32] respiration, immune function, energy metabolism, and growth. In most persons, blood copper levels are kept in a narrow range through the action of metallothionein (MT), ceruloplasmin, and other proteins. Unfortunately, many persons have a genetic inability to regulate copper levels and a serious copper overload can result.

Copper is a cofactor in the synthesis of norepinephrine, a neurotransmitter associated with several mental illnesses.[32] Norepinephrine is formed in the brain by the addition of a hydroxyl group to a dopamine molecule as shown in Figure 3-1. This reaction occurs in dopamine storage vesicles and is enabled by the enzyme dopamine β-hydroxylase (DBH) together with doubly-charged copper ions (Cu^{++}), vitamin C, and O_2 cofactors. DBH is a complex molecule containing 576 amino acids that binds to several copper ions. Vitamin C protects the DBH enzyme from oxidative reactions and supplies electrons for the reaction. The O_2 cofactor provides the oxygen atom for creation of the hydroxyl group.

Figure 3-1. Synthesis of Norepinephrine

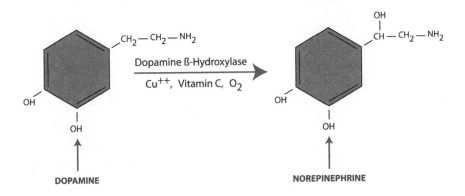

Copper overloads tend to lower dopamine levels and increase norepinephrine in the brain. Imbalances in these important neurotransmitters have been associated with paranoid schizophrenia, bipolar disorder, postpartum depression, ADHD, autism, and violent behavior. In two separate animal studies, a diet that lowered blood copper levels by 75% had a massive effect on norepinephrine and dopamine levels in the brain.[33-34]

Most persons with elevated blood copper also exhibit depressed zinc and excessive oxidative stress. In healthy persons, copper levels are regulated by MT and other proteins that bind to excess copper and carry it out of the body. However, MT activity can be significantly reduced by either zinc deficiency or elevated oxidative stress. Many persons diagnosed with mental illness have an inborn tendency for elevated copper levels, and this predisposes them to psychiatric disorders. Nutrient therapy to normalize copper levels can be effective in balancing dopamine and norepinephrine levels for these persons. This treatment approach is inexpensive and relatively free of side effects when administered properly.

Vitamin B-6 deficiency

Vitamin B-6 concentrations in the brain are about 100 times higher than levels in blood, and this nutrient has important roles in mental functioning. Severe deficiency of vitamin B-6[35-36] has been associated with irritability, depression, poor short-term memory, and psychosis. This is not surprising since it is required for efficient synthesis of serotonin,[37] dopamine,[38] and GABA,[39] three critically important neurotransmitters. There are three different chemical forms of B-6, the most common being pyridoxine hydrochloride, which converts to pyridoxal-5-phosphate (PLP, which is also known as P5P), the activated form of B-6 in the body and brain.

PLP is a strong aldehyde that has the ability to remove carboxyl groups (COOH) from molecules. An important example is the conversion of 5-HTP to serotonin (5-HT). Figure 3-2 shows the final step in the synthesis of serotonin that involves PLP as a coenzyme. In this reaction, PLP links to the enzyme aromatic L-amino-acid decarboxylase (AADC) and enables the removal of the OH- group from 5-HTP. Persons with a genetic or acquired B-6 deficiency tend to produce insufficient amounts of brain serotonin and are prone to clinical depression, OCD, and other mental problems. SSRI antidepressant medications, as an example, can increase serotonin activity in these persons, but nutrient therapy to normalize brain levels of vitamin B-6 and PLP may achieve the same result.

Vitamin B-6 in the form of PLP is also required for the synthesis of dopamine and GABA in the brain (Figures 3-3 and 3-4). A genetic or acquired deficiency of B-6 can result in abnormally low levels of these important neurotransmitters and a myriad of problems, including ADHD, depression, anxiety, and sleep disorders. A severe deficiency of B-6 can contribute to depressed levels of these neurotransmitters, resulting in mental disorders that are commonly treated with psychiatric medications

Figure 3-2. Synthesis of Serotonin

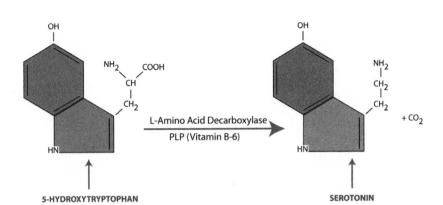

5-HYDROXYTRYPTOPHAN → SEROTONIN

L-Amino Acid Decarboxylase
PLP (Vitamin B-6)

$+ CO_2$

such as amphetamines, SSRIs, or benzodiazapines (e.g., Xanax). Vitamin therapy to normalize B-6 levels can provide treatment benefits and, in some cases, may eliminate the need for medication altogether.

In addition to the production of neurotransmitters, vitamin B-6 is involved in more than 80 biochemical reactions in the body. Vitamin B-6 deficiency can result in a wide variety of physical symptoms that are often vague and difficult to diagnose. These may include nervousness, insomnia, muscle weakness, and difficulty walking. The gold standard test for B-6 status is the transaminase stimulation blood test.[40]

Figure 3-3. Synthesis of Dopamine

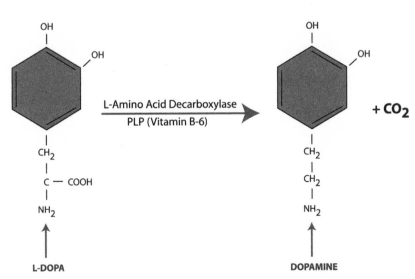

L-DOPA → DOPAMINE

L-Amino Acid Decarboxylase
PLP (Vitamin B-6)

$+ CO_2$

Figure 3-4. Synthesis of GABA

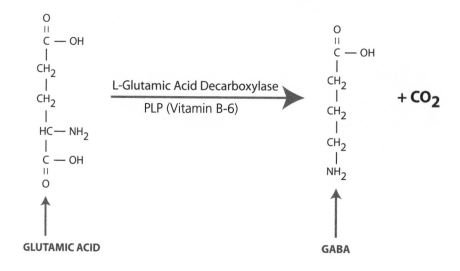

However, most B-6 deficient persons exhibit elevated pyrroles that can be detected by an inexpensive urine test.[27] Since B-6 deficiency is often caused by genetics, very high dosages may be necessary to normalize levels in the bloodstream and brain.

Overdoses of B-6 can cause neuropathy with loss of sensation in areas of the skin. However, this side effect is temporary and can be reversed by reducing B-6 intake. Another common symptom of B-6 overload is the onset of extremely troubling dreams. Persons who have a tendency for B-6 deficiency may tolerate very high dosages, but persons with B-6 sufficiency may react adversely to modest doses. In the mid-1980s, Dr. Carl Pfeiffer and I discovered that many slender malabsorbers diagnosed with schizophrenia failed to respond to the standard form of B-6 (pyridoxine hydrochloride) but improved significantly after receiving supplements of PLP. We later found that other patients responded better to the standard form of B-6. By the late 1980s, we began using a combination of standard B-6 together with PLP that appeared to benefit nearly all types of B-6 deficient patients, and this practice is still in use today.

Zinc deficiency

Zinc is a trace metal essential to all forms of life.[41] Most healthy human beings receive all the zinc they need from their diet. Absorption is usually very efficient, with about 38% of zinc in foods passing into the bloodstream. This dietary zinc is transported to the liver by albumin, transferrin, and L-histidine proteins in the portal bloodstream.

Once in the liver, most of the zinc is converted to zinc metallothionein that acts as a chaperone carrying zinc to cells throughout the body. Zinc is quite nontoxic when bound to a protein, and cases of zinc overload and poisoning are extremely rare.

Zinc deficiency is by far the most frequently observed chemical imbalance in mental health populations. More than 90% of persons diagnosed with depression, behavioral disorders, ADHD, autism, and schizophrenia exhibit depleted plasma zinc levels, ranging from low-normal to severe deficiency. One explanation for this curious fact is that most mental disorders involve oxidative stresses (described in Appendix B) that deplete zinc stores in the body. In addition, zinc has a special role in activation and inhibition of NMDA receptors that are essential to good mental health.

Zinc deficiency has been associated with delayed growth, temper control problems, poor immune function, depression, poor wound healing, epilepsy, anxiety, neurodegenerative disorders, hormone imbalances, and learning problems. Zinc is a component of more than 200 enzymes and is present in RNA polymerase, zinc fingers, and other special proteins that have key roles in cell division and genetic expression. Zinc has many important roles in brain function, which include the following:

- Zinc metallothionein is a key component of the blood-brain barrier that prevents harmful chemicals from entering the brain.
- Zinc proteins in the brain combat oxidative free radicals that could destroy brain cells, harm the myelin sheath, and alter neurotransmitter levels.
- Zinc is required for the efficient conversion of dietary B-6 into PLP, which is needed for efficient synthesis of serotonin, dopamine, GABA, and other neurotransmitters.
- Zinc deficiency can cause copper overloads that can alter brain levels of dopamine and norepinephrine.
- Zinc deficiency results in altered brain levels of GABA.
- Zinc is a neurotransmitter that is stored in vesicles and ejected into synapses.
- Zinc has a special role in the activation and inhibition of NMDA receptors.

Genetic or acquired zinc deficiency can usually be corrected within two months using nutrient therapy. This treatment must be done gradually for persons exhibiting serious overloads of toxic metals or copper in order to prevent temporary blood elevation of toxins as they depart the body. Increasing blood zinc levels results in higher production of MT and other zinc-bearing proteins that drive toxins out of the body. Special caution must be taken for persons with a cadmium overload since rapid removal can damage kidney tubules.

Many neuroscientists regard zinc as unimportant in mental illness for the following reasons:

♦ Most persons receive sufficient zinc from their diet.
♦ Homeostatic processes regulate blood zinc levels in most humans.
♦ Zinc is not directly involved in rate-controlling steps in the synthesis of most neurotransmitters.

However, millions of persons are born with a genetic tendency for severe zinc depletion that can disrupt brain chemistry and mental functioning. In working with thousands of violent children, we learned that most families report significant improvement once zinc levels are normalized. I believe lab testing for plasma zinc should be mandatory for all patients diagnosed with a behavioral disorder, ADHD, autism, or a mental illness.

Methyl/folate imbalances

In the 1960s, Abram Hoffer and colleagues proposed an adenochrome theory to explain auditory hallucinations. In the 1970s, Carl Pfeiffer published a theory that abnormal concentrations of brain histamine were responsible for paranoid schizophrenia and delusional disorders. In each case, subsequent research has failed to support the proposed theory. Medical history provides many examples of therapies that were highly effective many years before the correct scientific explanation was known.

My clinical experience with thousands of patients revealed the powerful impact of methylation status on several mental disorders.[42] I learned that low-serotonin depressives thrive on methylating agents such as methionine or SAMe but are intolerant to folates. In contrast, patients with excessive activity of dopamine and norepinephrine (for example, classic paranoid schizophrenia) thrive on folic acid and react adversely to SAMe and methionine. For years I was perplexed by the well-known fact that folic acid supplements increase methylation. The question has been "Why are undermethylated mentally ill patients intolerant to folates?" I spent many fruitless years investigating the impact of methyl and folates on neurotransmitter synthesis, including genetic expression of enzymes needed for neurotransmitter production. Eventually, I learned that the solution to this mystery lies in epigenetics and the factors that promote or inhibit gene expression of transporters at the synapse.

Mainstream psychiatry learned decades ago that drug treatments aimed at normalizing levels of brain chemicals such as serotonin, dopamine, etc. were relatively slow and ineffective. In contrast, medications that impact neurotransmitter activities at synapses were much more potent.[43] In early studies of depression, considerable attention was given to inhibiting proteins that destroy (metabolize) serotonin in the synapse. Monoamine oxidase is an enzyme that breaks down serotonin, and MAOI medications have been prescribed for depression since the 1970s. However, brain scientists eventually learned that the dominant factor at the synapse is the action of transporters, the special proteins that sweep neurotransmitters away from the synapse and return them back into the original brain cell. This reuptake process, previously introduced in Chapter 1, is the dominant factor at serotonin, dopamine, and norepinephrine synapses. This has been the basis for SSRI antidepressants, which bind to transporters and inactivate them.

There is little doubt that antidepressants can alleviate clinical depression in low-serotonin individuals. However, certain nutrient factors also can powerfully impact serotonin activity, and individualized nutrient therapy has the potential for normalizing serotonin activity and eliminating depression without significant side effects.

Abnormalities in methylation and folate chemistry are common in schizophrenia, bipolar disorder, depression, anxiety, and certain behavioral disorders.[44] Nearly all low-serotonin depressives tend to be deficient in methionine and SAMe and react adversely to folic acid. In another example, high-dopamine schizophrenics respond nicely to folate therapy and deteriorate if treated with SSRIs or non-folate methylating supplements. This curious phenomenon results from the epigenetic impact of methyl and folates on the production of transporters that control synaptic activity. As described in Chapter 4, folate deficiency results in reduced production of transporters and elevated synaptic activity. Undermethylation has the opposite effect, resulting in excessive gene expression of transporters and reduced synaptic activity.

With respect to mental health, the nutrient SAMe is a natural reuptake inhibitor for serotonin, dopamine, and norepinephrine. Folic acid is a natural reuptake enhancer that can combat excessive dopamine activity. The individual levels of methyl and folate in the brain are not as important as the methyl/folate ratio. Genetic or acquired imbalances in methyl and folate may be responsible for more than 50% of all mental illness. Psychiatric drugs may produce benefits for these persons, but nutrient therapy to balance methyl and folate levels provides a more scientific and direct approach that can avoid unpleasant side effects.

Nutrient therapy to normalize methyl and folate levels has resulted in thousands of reports of great improvement in patients afflicted by psychosis, depression, anxiety, and other illnesses. However, anecdotal case histories are poorly regarded by medical and scientific experts, and double-blind, placebo-controlled studies to measure treatment effectiveness will be necessary before this treatment approach can be embraced by mainstream psychiatry.

Oxidative stress

The role of oxidative stress in schizophrenia was first noticed when researchers in the 1960s observed elevated pyrrole levels in these patients. Pyrrole is a natural organic chemical containing a five-membered ring with the formula C_4H_4NH.[45] The term pyrrole is also used for several organic compounds containing a pyrrole ring. Pyrroles are involved in the synthesis of heme, the primary constituent of hemoglobin. Except for a role in the production of biochemicals, pyrroles are of minor importance and are efficiently excreted in urine. They have an affinity for binding with PLP and zinc, resulting in these valuable nutrients being transported out of the body together with the pyrroles. This process is a normal phenomenon for all human beings. However, some persons have a genetic (or acquired) tendency for very elevated levels of pyrroles, which can result in a deficiency of both PLP and zinc.

The alteration of neurotransmitter levels and mental functioning resulting from deficiency of either B-6 or zinc was described earlier in this chapter. Since pyrrole disorders involve simultaneous deficiency of both nutrients, behavioral and physical symptoms are generally more severe in this population. Classic symptoms of pyrrole disorder include high anxiety, frequent mood swings, poor short-term memory, reading disorder, morning nausea, absence of dream recall, and frequent anger and rages.

My colleagues and I have evaluated more than 40,000 urine pyrrole results for persons with a mental illness. Table 3-1 presents the incidence of elevated urine pyrroles (greater than 20 mcg/dl) in different clinical populations. As seen in the table, the incidence of pyrrole disorders is much higher in psychiatric disorders than in the general population. Most mental disorders involve oxidative stress, and elevated pyrroles may be secondary to a number of other biochemical conditions. However, psychiatric symptoms often recede or disappear after B-6 and zinc therapy and normalization of pyrrole levels. A genetic pyrrole disorder can result in low serotonin and GABA levels, and SSRI antidepressants and anti-anxiety medications often provide significant benefits. However, as is the case with other examples we've cited, nutrient therapy to normalize B-6 and zinc levels may provide similar benefits without unpleasant side effects.

Persons born with pyrrole disorder may have a lifetime tendency for deficiencies of B-6, zinc, and for high oxidative stress. A complication is that any source of oxidative stress can elevate urinary pyrrole levels. Many persons have elevated pyrroles resulting

Table 3-1.
Incidence of Pyrrole Overload in Clinical Populations

ADHD	18 %
Behavioral Disorder	28 %
Autism	35 %
Depression	24 %
Bipolar Disorder	35 %
Schizophrenia	30 %
Post-Traumatic Stress	12 %
Alzheimer's Disease	14 %
Healthy Controls	8 %

from factors such as physical accidents, illnesses, infections, emotional trauma, and toxic metals. Oxidative overloads from any source can cause psychosis in sensitive individuals by lowering glutamate neurotransmitter activity at NMDA receptors in the brain. Oxidative stresses deplete levels of glutathione (GSH) needed for efficient NMDA function. In schizophrenia, the term *oxidative stress overload* is more general and descriptive than the descriptors *pyroluria, mauve factor,* and *pyrrole disorder.* Biochemical markers for this condition include elevated urine pyrroles, low plasma zinc, depressed serum glutathione, elevated non-ceruloplasmin serum copper, and many others.

Amino acid disorders

A number of amino acids have important roles in brain chemistry.[44] Most human beings receive ample amounts of these amino acids from dietary protein and have proper concentrations in the brain. However, there are genetic errors that can alter the amounts of these chemicals in the brain and adversely impact mental functioning. Fortunately, this is a relatively rare occurrence. The roles of amino acids in brain chemistry are summarized below:

♦ Tryptophan is the initial starting point (substrate) for the synthesis of serotonin. For many years, tryptophan supplements have been used in an attempt to increase serotonin levels in the brain.

- Dopamine and norepinephrine are synthesized from either phenylalanine or tyrosine, and supplements of these amino acids may assist in elevating levels of these neurotransmitters.
- Glutamine is an amino acid that is a substrate for glutamic acid and the neurotransmitter GABA.
- GABA is both an amino acid and a neurotransmitter, and depressed levels have been associated with anxiety, depression, and psychosis.
- Aspartate is the starting point for the synthesis of the neurotransmitter aspartic acid.
- L-histidine is a precursor of the neurotransmitter histamine.
- Methionine is the precursor for SAMe that has a strong influence on genetic expression of several enzymes required for neurotransmitter synthesis and reuptake.

Fatty acid imbalance

There are more than 300 different fats in the human body, and the brain has a very high fat content (about 65%). Unsaturated fatty acids are especially important because they provide fluidity to cell membranes and assist in communication between brain cells. At brain synapses where the action is, four fats make up more than 90% of the lipid content: docosahexaenoic acid (DHA), eicosapentaenoic acid (EPA), arachidonic acid (AA), and dihomo-gamma-linolenic acid (DGLA). Of these, DHA (an omega-3 fatty acid) is found in the highest concentration and appears to have the greatest impact on brain function. DHA deficiency has been associated with depression, ADHD, schizophrenia, bipolar disorder, and dementia. Second in importance may be EPA, another omega-3 fatty acid. DHA and EPA are essential fatty acids (EFAs) that have become very popular nutritional supplements. Seafood and fish oils are excellent omega-3 dietary sources. AA and DGLA are omega-6 EFAs and are at excessive levels in most persons who consume a junk food diet. The ideal proportion of EFAs in the diet is considered by nutritionists to be between 3 and 6 grams of omega-6 for each gram of omega-3. Unfortunately, a typical American diet contains an excessive amount of omega-6 and other unhealthy fats.

Because of genetic variations, there is biochemical individuality with respect to the ideal dietary intake of specific fatty acids, and indiscriminant use of omega-3 supplements could worsen symptoms for certain patients. For example, most persons with severe pyrrole disorder have sufficient levels of omega-3 oils but are very deficient in AA. In my experience, these patients thrive on primrose oil, which is rich in omega-6; however, they may deteriorate if they supplement with omega-3 alone. In contrast, most depressives and schizophrenics are deficient in DHA and EPA and thrive on omega-3 supplements.

Most mental disorders involve elevated oxidative stress that can be quite lethal to EFAs. Fortunately, phosphatidyls are fatty acids that provide a safe haven for DHA, EPA, AA, and DGLA in the presence of oxidative free radicals. The four major phosphatidyls have choline, serine, inositol, or ethanolamine attached to the end of the molecule. Several phosphotidyls are available commercially and can assist in combating certain mental illnesses.

Glucose dysregulation

Our database indicates a significant number of patients exhibit chronic low blood glucose levels. This problem doesn't appear to be the cause of behavioral disorders or mental illnesses, but it is instead an aggravating factor that can trigger striking symptoms. Typical symptoms include drowsiness after meals, irritability, craving for sweets, trembling, anxiety, and intermittent poor concentration and focus. Treatment includes chromium, manganese, and other glucose-stabilizing nutrients, but the primary focus of treatment is on diet. These patients benefit from six or more small meals daily with emphasis on complex carbohydrates and protein. In essence, they cannot tolerate large meals or quick sugars. Complex carbohydrates provide the necessary glucose in a slow, gradual manner and may be thought of as timed-release sugar.

Toxic overload

My database includes many patients who exhibit elevated levels of toxic metals, pesticides, or other organic chemicals. Overloads of lead, mercury, and cadmium are especially common. Persons with depressed levels of zinc, glutathione, selenium, or metallothionein are especially sensitive to toxic metals. A high percentage of overmethylated mental patients exhibit severe sensitivities to pesticides and toxic industrial chemicals. Effective treatment of a toxic overload requires a three-part approach:

- Avoidance of additional exposures
- Biochemical treatment to hasten the exit of the toxins from the body
- Correction of underlying chemical imbalances to minimize future vulnerability to toxins

Malabsorption

Although only 10% of mental illness cases involve serious malabsorption, more than

90% of autistics exhibit this problem. There are three primary classes of absorption problems:

- Stomach problems, including excessive or insufficient levels of hydrochloric acid
- Incomplete digestion in the small intestine
- Problems at the brush-border of the intestine where most nutrients are absorbed into the portal blood stream

The consequences can include nutrient deficiencies, inflammation in the intestinal tract, *Candida*, and many other gastrointestinal (GI) disorders. Incomplete breakdown of protein and fats can cause physical problems and also adversely affect brain function. Elevated oxidative stress can destroy digestive enzymes needed for processing protein and is a frequent cause of malabsorption. A high percentage of malabsorbing patients have a compromised and, thus, ineffective intestinal barrier, allowing toxic metals and other undesirable substances to enter the body and access the brain. Treatment depends on the type of malabsorption present and may involve the adjustment of stomach acid levels, administration of digestive enzymes that survive stomach acid, administration of antioxidants, and use of special diets.

Other Nutrient Imbalances
Many other nutrients play a significant role in mental functioning. Selenium, vitamin C, vitamin E, and other natural antioxidants combat inflammation and free radicals in the brain and indirectly increase glutamate activity at NMDA receptors. Vitamin D deficiency has been associated with depression, schizophrenia, ADHD, and other mental disorders. Vitamin D levels increase during exposure to sunlight, and it's not a surprise that northern Scandinavia, with its relatively low amount of sunlight, has an extremely high incidence of schizophrenia.

The Interface with Psychiatric Medication
Most schizophrenic patients are taking psychiatric medication at the time of the first appointment and express a desire to discontinue the drugs. However, the medication usually has produced definite benefits, and we urge continued compliance during the initial stages of biochemical therapy. If clear progress is achieved after several months of both therapies together, then we suggest the family return to their psychiatrist for a cautious trial of reduced medication dosages. The goal is *not* to eliminate psychiatric medication but to identify the dosage needed for maximum benefits.

Our internal outcome studies indicate that more than 70% of behavior, ADHD, and depression patients report they are at their best with zero medication after six months of biochemical therapy. The remaining 30% state that some medication support is needed to prevent a partial return of symptoms. In nearly all cases, medication dosages can safely be reduced with lessened side effects. The situation is very different for patients diagnosed with schizophrenia or bipolar disorder, with only 5% able to completely discontinue psychiatric medication after successful biochemical therapy. Many of these patients report elimination of psychosis and a return to independent living after a combination of nutrient therapy and greatly reduced medication levels. Reduction of side effects often increases a patient's willingness to take medication and eliminates the dire consequences that can result from sudden noncompliance. In general, psychiatric medications appear to be much more effective after nutrient imbalances have been corrected. The two therapeutic approaches clearly are in harmony with each other.

For the past several decades, treatment of mental illness has focused on imbalanced brain chemistry and the use of drugs to alter the activity of serotonin, dopamine, and other neurotransmitters. Back in 1970, drugs were the only method known to have a powerful impact on molecular processes in the brain. This approach proved to be highly successful and has benefited millions of persons diagnosed with depression, schizophrenia, ADHD and other mental disorders. However, science has made great advances in the understanding of complex brain processes, and we are approaching an era in which psychiatric medications may no longer be necessary. It is time to move aggressively in the development of epigenetic therapies and other advanced techniques that have the potential to normalize brain function without drugs or significant adverse side effects.

Nutrient Therapy Response Times

Nutrient therapy can have a powerful impact on mental functioning, but several weeks or months are usually needed to achieve the full effect. In contrast, most psychiatric medications can affect symptoms within a few hours or days. For example, SSRI antidepressants quickly bind to transporters, resulting in a rapid increase in serotonin activity at the synapse. Methylation therapy for depression using SAMe or methionine reduces genetic expression of transporters, resulting in a slow and gradual increase in serotonin activity over a period of several months. In another example, nutrient therapy to eliminate copper overloads in the blood usually requires about 60 days.

The chemical imbalance with the fastest response is pyrrole disorder, with significant progress often reported during the first week. This rapid response results from the ability to normalize vitamin B-6 levels in a short time. Zinc deficiency usually can be corrected within 60 days. Treatment of overmethylation usually entails no improvement the first two weeks, with gradual progress over the next four to eight weeks. Undermethylation is the slowest chemical imbalance to resolve, with three to nine months often required for the full effect. Patients should be informed of the expected treatment time frame associated with biochemical treatments so they won't become discouraged by lack of immediate progress.

The Value of Counseling

I've encountered thousands of depressed and psychotic patients who have received major benefits from counseling. Psychodynamic therapies not only provide insight, coping mechanisms, and self-image repair, but also can have an enduring impact on gene expression. There is evidence that effective counseling can also promote development of new synapses and neuronal minicolumns, thereby permanently improving the microstructure of the brain. Correcting brain chemistry often is not enough, and counseling can enhance the benefits patients can enjoy. For example, behavior-disordered teens may have a negative self-image and poor habits that cannot be corrected by chemistry alone. Many anorexic patients have reported nice improvement from nutrient therapies but needed effective counseling to achieve complete recovery. Nutrient therapy and counseling are natural partners.

Chemical Classification of Mental Illnesses

Over the past 20 years, psychiatry has achieved remarkable progress in the understanding of complex brain processes. However, development of improved treatments for depression, schizophrenia, and other illnesses has been hindered by the failure to separate these disorders into meaningful phenotypes. Depression is an umbrella term used to describe a collection of disorders that have very different brain chemistries, symptoms, and traits. The same thing is true for the terms schizophrenia, bipolar disorder, and ADHD. For example, some depressives have low serotonin activity, but others exhibit elevated serotonin activity. SSRIs, the serotonin-enhancing medications, have shown efficacy for mixed groups of depressives because more than 50% of the depressives have low activity of this neurotransmitter. However, more than 30% of depressives are not low-serotonin patients, and for them an SSRI will likely be either neutral or harmful. The most common phenotype of schizophrenia involves elevated dopamine activity, and most current antipsychotic medications are aimed at lowering activity of this neurotransmitter. Unfortunately, this is the wrong approach for schizophrenics with different brain chemistry. Most efficacy experiments for depression and schizophrenia continue to involve a mixture of disorders with different brain chemistry imbalances. This blurs the data and weakens the scientific findings. Some psychiatry experts have recently urged researchers to develop objective tests for separating these illnesses into meaningful phenotypes.

This book presents biochemical classifications for depression and schizophrenia based on (a) more than one million blood and urine chemical assays, and (b) identification of distinctive symptoms and traits for each chemical type. To the extent possible with present knowledge, I have indicated the primary neurotransmitter imbalances for each of the depression and schizophrenia phenotypes in the following chapters. This technology can help psychiatrists identify promising psychiatric medications for different patients through inexpensive blood/urine testing. This information also provides a roadmap for the development of nutrient therapies for these disorders.

CHAPTER 4

EPIGENETICS AND MENTAL HEALTH

Introduction

The new science of epigenetics[46-47] has revolutionized our understanding of the brain and is leading to exciting breakthroughs in treatment of mental illnesses. Epigenetics is a rapidly growing field that investigates alterations in gene expression that do not involve changes in DNA sequence. Until recently, a person's genetic characteristics were thought to be cast in concrete at the moment of conception, with a unique DNA sequence arising from a somewhat random collection of genetic factors from parents and ancestors. We now know this is only partially true and that the chemical environment in the womb can determine which genes are expressed and which are silenced in the various tissues and organs. In addition, environmental factors can alter genetic expression throughout life.

Many mental disorders result from environmental factors that cause genes to behave (or express themselves) improperly.[48] For example, nutrient imbalances or toxic exposures can alter gene expression rates and may be the root cause of numerous psychiatric disorders. It's not a coincidence that methylation is a dominant factor in epigenetics, and methylation abnormalities are common in mental illnesses. Recent advances in the science of epigenetics provide a roadmap for nutrient therapies that have potential for overcoming mental disorders and eventual elimination of the need for psychiatric medications.

Epigenetics 101

All cells in the human body contain an identical copy of DNA with the potential for producing more than 20,000 proteins. However, the proteins needed in liver cells are different from those of skin cells, pancreas cells, and so on. Epigenetics provides the blueprint that specifies the combination of proteins to be manufactured in each tissue.[49] Without epigenetics, we could be an amorphous blob of identical cells instead of an organism with arms, eyeballs, teeth, and other diverse parts. Certain nutrients have a powerful role in determining which genes are expressed or silenced in different tissues, and proper balance between these nutrient factors is essential for good mental health.

DNA consists of billions of proteins that form a double-helix ribbon that would be about six feet in length if stretched out. This DNA is amazingly packed into a tiny ball that is about one-hundredth of a millimeter in diameter and neatly fits inside the nucleus of every cell. This fragile double helix is wrapped around tiny globs of protein called histones in a configuration known as beads on a string. The acidic DNA strand gently adheres to millions of histones which are slightly alkaline. The histone-DNA beads are called nucleosomes,[50] and an array of nucleosomes is termed chromatin. Figure 4-1 is a schematic of a nucleosome. A histone consists of eight linear proteins clumped together like a ball of yarn, with several protein tails protruding from the array. The DNA ribbon wraps around each of the millions of histones slightly less than two times (146 base pairs). For years, scientists believed histones provided a support framework for the fragile DNA but did not have a role in gene expression. Researchers recently established that genes can be turned on or off, depending on which chemicals react with the histone tails. Abnormal histone modifications are common in mental illness,[51-52] and nutrient therapy can assist in normalizing histone chemistry.

The two dominant epigenetic processes are DNA methylation[53] and histone modification[54] as shown in Fig. 4-2. DNA methylation involves addition of methyl groups to some of the cytosine molecules along the double helix. In most cases, methylation in the vicinity of a gene tends to silence expression of that gene. This process is a crucial part of human development that helps determine which proteins are

Figure 4-1. Schematic of a Nucleosome

DNA

HISTONE TAILS

8 HISTONE CORE

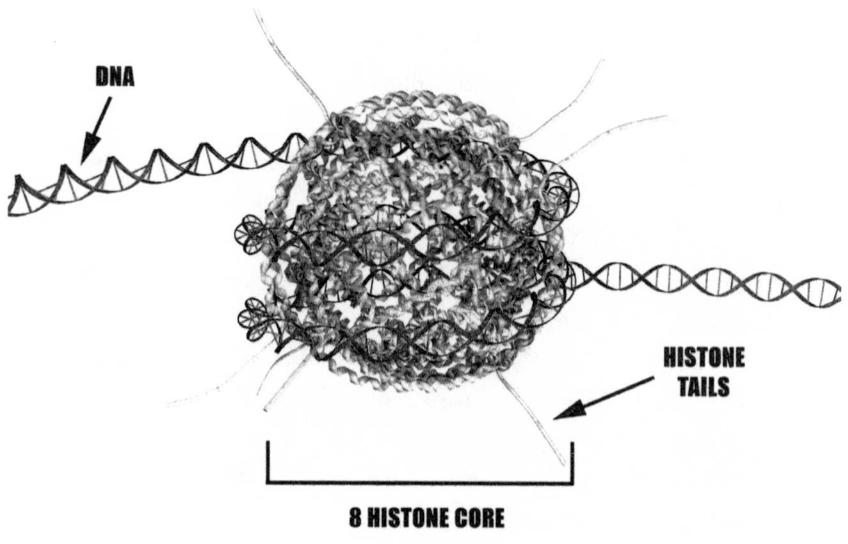

produced in different tissues and organs. DNA methylation also prevents expression of viruses and other junk genes that have been implicated in disease conditions.

In many cases, genetic expression depends on competition between acetyl and methyl groups at histone tails. If tails are predominantly acetylated, genetic expression

Figure 4-2. The Two Main Components of the Epigenetic Code

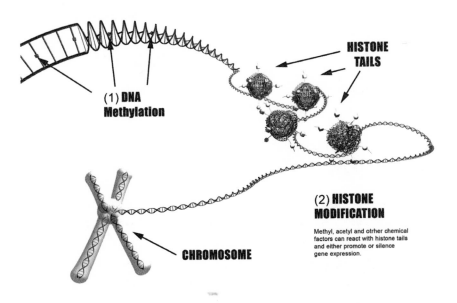

(protein production) is promoted. In contrast, highly methylated histones generally result in silencing of genetic expression. Many scientists believe that the ability to express genes is determined by the degree of compactness of chromatin as illustrated in Figures 4-3 and 4-4. This theory recognizes that acetyl groups lower the pH of alkaline histones, thus reducing the electrostatic attraction to DNA and allowing the array to open up and promote genetic expression. Methyl groups produce the opposite effect by increasing compactness of chromatin and silencing genetic expression.

After conception, all of the methyl, acetyl, and other regulating chemicals from the parents' DNA are removed from the DNA of the fetus and a new set of chemicals attached during early fetal development. These chemicals are called bookmarks (or marks) since they regulate the expression of every gene and can remain in place through a lifetime of cell divisions. Deviant marks that develop in utero can result in a variety of diseases and developmental disorders. Most deviant marks associated with mental illnesses are believed to involve inappropriate placement of methyl and acetyl groups on DNA or histone tails.

Figure 4-3. Low Methylation Promotes Gene Expression

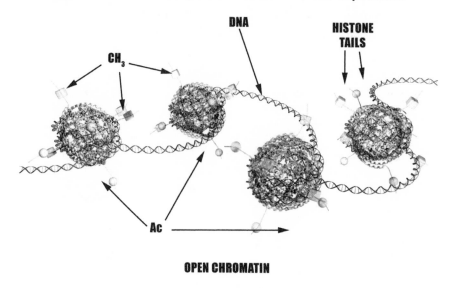

Histone epigenetics is proving to be extraordinarily complex, and it may take another century to completely describe the processes involved. A total of 69 different histone proteins have been identified, each with different chemical characteristics. Acetyl and methyl levels dominate the expression/silencing of many genes, but other chemical factors such as phosphate, biotin, ubiquitin, and citrullin can react with histones and influence gene expression.[55] In addition, special enzymes called

Figure 4-4. High Methylation Inhibits Gene Expression

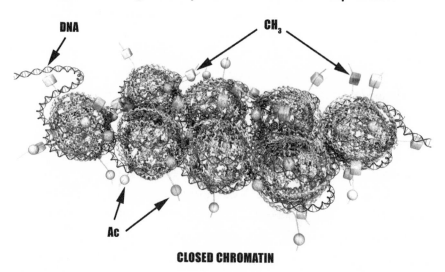

transcription factors are recruited by specific combinations of histone proteins and reactants and interact with the local DNA to influence cell expression. There may be more than 2,000 transcription factors, indicating there are a great multitude of different histone reactions that can occur. A complex histone code is under development.

Transcription factors

Gene expression requires separation (or uncoiling) of DNA from histones to allow certain large molecules to access areas near that gene. The process of gene transcription (copying of DNA by RNA polymerase into RNA) requires the presence of one or more transcription factors[56] (complex proteins such as zinc fingers). Transcription factors are proteins that bind to specific areas of DNA and regulate the access of RNA polymerase (the enzyme that performs the transcription of genetic information from DNA to RNA). A defining feature of transcription factors is that they contain one or more DNA-binding domains, which attach to specific sequences of DNA adjacent to the genes that they regulate.

There are more than 2,500 proteins in the human genome that have DNA-binding domains, and most are assumed to function as transcription factors. Some transcription factors promote gene expression, while others are inhibitory. The enormous diversity of these proteins may be essential to development of in utero tissue differentiation. They have several mechanisms, including regulation of acetyl and methyl levels at CpG islands (genomic regions that contain a high frequency of cytosine-phosphate-guanine sites) and histones. It is very likely that many nutrients have an impact on transcription factors, but these relationships are poorly understood at present.

The Methyl-Acetyl Competition

Methyl groups are delivered to histones by SAMe and acetyl groups by acetyl coenzyme A. Both of these chemical factors are in high concentration throughout the entire body. SAMe is a natural protein produced in the liver from dietary methionine. SAMe provides methyl groups for dozens of important biochemical reactions in the body and is conserved by a process called the methylation cycle or one-carbon cycle.[57] Acetyl coenzyme A is formed from the metabolism (breakdown) of protein, fats, and carbohydrates and delivers high-energy acetyl groups to the mitochondria for processing in the citric acid cycle. Both acetyl and methyl are essential to life.

Attachment or removal of methyl and acetyl at histone tails is dominated by enzymes called methylases, acetylases, demethylases, and deacetylases—NOT by the amounts of methyl and acetyl present. There is considerable research aimed at developing drugs that can regulate the relative amounts of these enzymes. However, certain nutrients have a powerful effect on these enzymes and epigenetic nutrient therapies may be equally effective. A good example[58] is niacinamide (vitamin B-3) that reduces the activity of sirtuin, an important deacetylase enzyme. In another example,[59] folic acid impacts methyl levels at histones. It's interesting to note that folates increase methyl levels in tissues and the bloodstream, but they reduce methylation at certain histones that regulate gene expression. It's clear that many nutrients have a powerful impact on gene expression and that epigenetic nutrient therapies have great promise.

Neurotransmitter Transporter Proteins

Neurotransmitter transporter proteins, also known as transporters (see Chapter 1), are transmembrane proteins that quickly remove neurotransmitter molecules from a synapse for reuse in future cell firings. Gene expression of serotonin, dopamine, and norepinephrine transporters is dominated by a competition between methyl and acetyl groups at the histone tails. If acetylation dominates, the production of transporters is increased and neurotransmitter activity is reduced. If methylation wins the battle, gene expression of transporters is inhibited, resulting in higher neurotransmitter activity. In essence, nutrients that promote histone methylation are natural serotonin reuptake inhibitors.

Placing acetyl groups on histones is enabled by enzymes called histone acetyltransferases (HATs).[60] Acetyl groups can be readily removed by chemicals called histone deacetylases (HDACs). Several HAT and HDAC enzymes have been identified. Enzymes called histone methyltransferases (HMTs) promote the transfer of one to three methyl groups from SAMe to specific amino acid locations along the linear histone proteins. For many years, histone methylation was thought to be a permanent modification. Very recently, two families of histone demethylating enzymes were discovered. Nutrients or drugs that promote or inhibit expression of these enzymes can have a major impact on neurotransmitter reuptake and synaptic activity.

Epigenetics and Brain Functioning

Healthy mental functioning requires a proper level of synaptic activity at receptors for serotonin, dopamine, norepinephrine, and other neurotransmitters. Proper synaptic activity depends on:

◆   The amount of neurotransmitter produced in brain cells

♦ The amount of synaptic neurotransmitters lost by diffusion or reaction with chemicals
♦ The availability of transporters that return synaptic neurotransmitters back into the original brain cell (reuptake)

Decades of pharmaceutical research have shown that synaptic activity is dominated by the concentration of transporters. SSRI antidepressants,[61] such as Prozac and Zoloft, inactivate transporters to increase serotonin levels within synapses. SNRI medications, such as Effexor, use the same mechanism to increase activity of both serotonin and norepinephrine. In contrast, benzodiazapine medications, such as Xanax and Valium, increase GABA activity by directly binding to GABA receptors, thus reducing the impact of excessive norepinephrine activity. All three classes of these medications can provide impressive benefits in combating depression, anxiety, etc. but are very addictive and often cause troubling side effects such as fatigue, loss of libido, weight gain, and headaches, among others.

Epigenetics research has identified several nutrient factors that have a powerful impact on transporters at neurotransmitter synapses, including methionine, SAMe, folic acid, niacinanide, and zinc. These are the same nutrients pioneered by Hoffer, Pfeiffer, and the author that have produced thousands of reports of recovery from schizophrenia, depression, anxiety, ADHD, and behavioral disorders. It is highly unlikely that this is a coincidence. In addition, epigenetics research has identified several other nutrients with potential for improving brain functioning. Since nutrient therapy involves normalization of brain chemistry, this approach has the great advantage of minimal adverse side effects.

Two types of epigenetic disorders

Epigenetic disorders can result from either (a) fetal programming errors or (b) deviant gene bookmarks that develop later in life. In both cases, environmental insults are believed responsible for the deviant marks that can persist throughout the remainder of life. Fetal programming errors can result in developmental disorders that are evident from birth. However, deviant fetal programming may also produce predisposition for disorders that appear after birth such as cancer, heart disease, and regressive autism. Epigenetic disorders that appear before age three may result in brain structure abnormalities that are irreversible. In contrast, deviant epigenetic marks that cause brain chemistry imbalances are likely to be reversible. Future epigenetic therapies may eventually result in an enduring cure for anxiety, depression, schizophrenia, and other mental disorders.

Two types of epigenetic therapy

In theory, abnormal gene expression can be corrected either temporarily or permanently. Except for recent cancer research, all epigenetic treatments have been the temporary type in which gene expression rates are modified without changes in the marks. These treatments cause one of two outcomes: (1) uncoiling DNA from histones to enhance gene expression rates or (2) tighter compaction of DNA and histones to reduce expression rates. However, the resulting benefits in mental function can disappear if the treatments are stopped. Future therapies to permanently correct deviant marks could achieve a cure for several mental illnesses within a decade or two. The development of advanced epigenetic treatments should be a high national priority.

Epigenetics and Nutrient Therapy
Methionine and SAMe

Carl Pfeiffer developed a methylation therapy[28] for high-histamine schizophrenic patients that brought thousands of reports of improvement. Pfeiffer believed that histamine imbalances in the brain caused psychosis, and he prescribed methionine as a therapy to lower histamine levels in these patients. In the early 1990s, I discovered that histamine was relatively unimportant and that methyl status was a dominant factor in psychosis. Undermethylated persons were prone to depression that usually could be lessened by SSRIs. Overmethylated persons were prone to high-anxiety depression that usually worsened after SSRIs. Epigenetics has provided a clear insight into the importance of methylation therapy in mental health.[62-63] Methionine and SAMe increase histone methylation, which can inhibit gene expression of serotonin transport proteins. The result is increased serotonin in synapses and higher serotonin activity. In effect, methionine and SAMe are natural serotonin reuptake inhibitors.

Folic acid

Abram Hoffer pioneered the use of folic acid therapy for schizophrenia in the 1950s. About 10 years later, Pfeiffer found that most paranoid schizophrenics responded very well to folic acid supplements but that delusional schizoaffective patients deteriorated if given folic acid. My experience with thousands of schizophrenic patients confirmed Pfeiffer's folic acid observations. However, I became puzzled by the fact that folic acid is an effective methylating agent, but it has a negative effect on undermethylated schizophrenics and depressives. Overmethylated patients clearly thrive on folic acid, whereas methyl-deficient patients exhibit intolerance. In 1994, I reported this surprising finding at the Society for Neuroscience annual meeting[42] and concluded that the methyl/folate ratio has a special significance in mental health. Recent epigenetic research has finally provided a convincing explanation for this phenomenon. Several studies[64-66] have shown that **reducing** dietary folates can **increase** methylation at histone tails and DNA sites. Vanderbilt University biochemists have reported that folates enhance histone demethylation.[61] A National Institutes of Health (NIH) study reported that activation of a folic acid receptor gene can increase histone acetylation.[67] In effect, folic acid increases genetic expression of transporters, causing **reduced** activity of dopamine and serotonin. Folate and methyl produce opposite effects on neurotransmission. Folic acid is a serotonin reuptake enhancer, whereas methionine and SAMe are serotonin reuptake inhibitors. Giving folic acid to an undermethylated depression patient results in improved methyl levels (SAMe) throughout the body and brain but reduced methyl levels at key histones and CpG islands that regulate neurotransmitter activity.

Folic acid supplements can either increase or decrease methylation at histone tails and CpG islands, depending on the portion of the DNA strand that is involved. With respect to mental health, folic acid supplements generally must be avoided for undermethylated patients and emphasized for overmethylated patients.

Vitamin B-3 (niacin)

For many years, Abram Hoffer championed the use of niacin (vitamin B-3) in the treatment of schizophrenia. Later, Carl Pfeiffer reported that niacin was highly effective for patients with low blood histamine levels but less beneficial for others. In the early 1990s, I observed that niacinamide, the active form of niacin in the body, could be substituted for niacin in treatment of high-dopamine patients. After years of confusion and uncertainty, epigenetics has provided a convincing explanation for the efficacy of niacin. Niacinamide inhibits sirtuins, a class of proteins that effectively remove acetyl groups from histones and promote methylation.[58] By this mechanism, increased intake of vitamin B-3 (niacin or niacinamide) results in higher gene expression of transporters and reduced dopamine activity. This is especially useful for paranoid schizophrenics who have excessive dopamine activity.

Other nutrients

In addition to the powerful impacts of methyl, acetyl, folate, and niacin on brain chemistry, several other nutrients are known to influence the epigenetics of neurotransmission.[68] For example, biotin and phosphates can covalently bind to histones and impact gene expression. Zinc enhances the gene expression of metallothionein, an important antioxidant protein. Many other nutrients affect the production and functioning of enzymes and cofactors that govern epigenetic processes. Pantothenic acid, tryptophan, choline, and dimethylaminoethanol (DMAE) enhance acetylation of histones. In addition, various nutrients have an important impact on DNA promoter regions that regulate gene expression rates.

Identification of Epigenetic Disorders

In Chapter 3, I alluded to my work over the past 35 years, wherein I collected a database of more than three million blood, urine, and tissue chemistries from 30,000 patients diagnosed with a variety of mental disorders. Methylation status was assessed for each of these patients based on lab chemistries and medical history. I discovered that the incidence of a methylation disorder approaches 100% in certain psychiatric conditions. Since methyl status is a dominant factor in epigenetics, there is a strong possibility that these conditions are epigenetic in nature. This belief is supported by the fact that these disorders are heritable (run in families) but violate classical laws of Mendelian genetics with less than 100% concordance for identical twins.

An environmental insult that triggers an epigenetic illness would likely involve altered expression of several genes. As a result, epigenetic mental disorders would be expected to involve a consistent syndrome of symptoms and behavioral traits. For example, autism usually involves poor immune function; altered brain structure; digestive abnormalities; odd, repetitive movements; etc., all of which form a distinctive syndrome that is typical of an epigenetic disorder. The following disorders meet my criteria for an epigenetic disorder: abnormal methylation, non-Mendelian heritability, and a syndrome of distinctive symptoms and traits. However, the most convincing indicator of an epigenetic condition is a sudden onset followed by a permanent change in functioning. Since deviant marks survive many cell divisions, the condition doesn't just go away. Future epigenetic therapies aimed at correcting aberrant gene expression have great potential for benefitting these patients.

Autism: In 1999, Bernard Rimland of the Autism Research Institute learned that I had amassed the world's largest collection of chemistry data for autism spectrum children and asked me to identify any consistent abnormalities in this population. My data confirmed previous reports of disordered metal metabolism, B-6 deficiency, and elevated toxic metals, but the data also produced the surprising finding that more than 95% of autistics exhibited undermethylation. This has led to convincing research by S. Jill James,[69] Richard Deth,[70] and others, indicating that undermethylation is a distinctive feature of autism spectrum disorders. Both the autistic regression event and the persistence of autism symptoms are also consistent with a gene expression disorder. As described in Chapter 7, there is growing evidence that autism is epigenetic in nature.[71-72]

Schizoaffective disorder: This condition[73] is a mixed thought, mood, and perceptual disorder consisting of delusional thinking, moods ranging from depression to mania, and perceptual hallucinations and illusions. In most cases, delusional thinking is the dominant symptom. Many of these patients also exhibit obsessive-compulsive tendencies, internal anxiety, and catatonic tendencies. Typically, this is an adult-onset condition featuring a mental breakdown after a history of high achievement. A review of the chemistry database for 500 persons with this diagnosis revealed that virtually all had evidence of undermethylation. I believe this devastating disorder is epigenetic in nature.

Paranoid schizophrenia: This severe mental disorder[73] usually involves auditory hallucinations and paranoia along with a multitude of other troubling symptoms. Review of the database for more than 1,000 persons with this diagnosis revealed that more than 85% exhibited overmethylation. This condition is often misdiagnosed, and a careful study of 250 patients with classic symptoms indicated overmethylation in 94% of the patients. With more accurate diagnosis, the incidence of this chemical imbalance could approach 100%. A typical feature of this illness is a mental breakdown after age 15. It seems likely that classic paranoid schizophrenia is epigenetic in nature.

Obsessive-compulsive disorder (OCD): My chemistry database contains 92 individuals diagnosed with severe OCD.[73] Many reported that the condition appeared quite suddenly and has been a chronic problem since that time. All but five exhibited severe undermethylation. This strongly suggests that OCD is epigenetic in origin.

Antisocial personality disorder (ASPD): My behavior database includes chemistry information for more than 800 convicted felons and thousands of very violent children. Examination of data for more than 400 persons diagnosed with ASPD[73] indicated a high incidence of zinc deficiency, pyrrole disorder, toxic metal overload, and glucose dyscontrol. However, more than 96% also exhibited undermethylation, suggesting this condition may be epigenetic in origin and involve aberrant brain development and altered neurotransmitter activity. Future treatments that modify methyl and acetyl levels at histones and DNA CpG sites may represent an effective way to reduce crime and violence.

Anorexia: Examination of chemistry information for 145 persons diagnosed with anorexia[73] revealed that all but five were undermethylated. Nutrient therapy to enhance methylation together with counseling has produced many reports of recovery. This is another strong candidate for epigenetics research.

Paraphilias:[73] My chemistry database includes a few dozen persons with abnormal sexual behaviors including pedophiles, sexual sadists, masochists, and peeping toms. All of these patients were male and most were in trouble with the law. They complained of overwhelming intrusive thoughts that interfered with daily life. Only two said they had been sexually abused as children. In most cases, they first became aware of their condition between the ages of 14-16. More than 90% were undermethylated, suggesting that paraphilias may be epigenetic in origin. I believe that the term obsessive-compulsive perversion or OCP is more appropriate than paraphilia. It's well known that child molesters rarely reform regardless of medications, counseling interventions, or the threat of imprisonment. Perhaps future epigenetic therapies may rid the world of this devastating and criminal disorder.

Transgenerational Epigenetic Inheritance (TEI)

Animal experiments have clearly shown that certain epigenetic errors can be transmitted to future generations, without changing DNA sequence.[74] There is growing evidence that this mechanism also occurs in humans. This means that the harmful effects of a toxic exposure can be passed on to one's children and grandchildren. I'm reminded of a quotation from the Bible: "The sins of the father are visited upon the son." Imprinting of abnormal methylation of the genome is believed to be one of the major TEI mechanisms. We are all familiar with physical birth defects that can result from toxic exposures during pregnancy. TEI defects could also cause abnormal brain development, chemical imbalances, weakened immune function, and an inborn predisposition for a mental illness. In addition, TEI may have contributed to the mysterious recent epidemics in ADHD, autism, breast cancer, and other conditions that have a strong heritable component.

Nature, Nurture, and Epigenetics

For centuries, scientists have debated whether mental illness results from inborn or environmental factors. At long last, these arguments are fading away as most experts now agree that both factors are highly important. Schizophrenia and many other mental illnesses involve inherited predispositions but violate classic laws of Mendelian genetics, thereby indicating a strong influence of environment. The new science of epigenetics has shown that gene expression can go awry due to toxic chemicals, emotional trauma, chronic personal failures, oxidative stress, medication side effects, nuclear radiation, and abnormal nutrient levels. The good news is that deviant gene marks may be normalized by future epigenetic therapies. Present epigenetics research is focused on the development of drugs that can alter gene expression, but epigenetic nutrient therapies may be equally effective.

The initial book chapters have summarized the basic facts and overarching principles needed to understand underlying chemical imbalances in the brain associated with mental illnesses as well as other conditions encompassing cognitive deficits. We have shown, in a general sense, how nutrients can often accomplish what drugs hope to achieve but in a more natural manner that is less prone to adverse side effects. The remaining chapters will focus on schizophrenia, depression, autism spectrum disorders, behavioral disorders, and Alzheimer's disease. Some information that we've included in the preceding chapters is, by necessity, included, and we hope this serves to reinforce key points to the reader.

CHAPTER 5

SCHIZOPHRENIA

Introduction

Schizophrenia was first described by the ancient Egyptians[75] and has remained an enigma throughout recorded history. It is an equal-opportunity disease that afflicts approximately 0.3% of all human beings and is found in all geographical areas, ethnic groups, and economic classes. It is a broad term used to describe a collection of completely different mental disorders. Schizophrenia typically develops between the ages of 15-25 for males and 16-35 for females. The symptoms, especially hallucinations, delusions, paranoia, and radical changes in personality, are usually quite shocking to family and friends. In most cases, the net result is a lifetime of misery for the patient, mental anguish and depleted finances for the family, and a great public sacrifice in terms of lost human potential and increased national health care costs.

A Brief History of Schizophrenia

Written documents describing schizophrenia extend back to 2,000 B.C. The condition was generally referred to as madness until the 19th century, and the cause was generally assumed to be possession by evil spirits. In the Middle Ages, popular treatments included (a) exorcism of the demons in a religious ceremony and (b) releasing evil spirits by drilling holes in the patient's skull.

Schizophrenia was first recognized as a mental illness in the 1800s. The French psychiatrist Falvet[76] described a *folie circulaire* or cyclical madness in 1851, and German psychiatrist Ewald Hecker[77] referred to a hebephrenia or a silly, undisciplined mind in 1871. Karl Kahlbaum[78] described both catatonic and paranoid disorders in 1874. A major milestone in psychiatry was made in 1896 by Emil Kraepelin[79] of Germany, who combined these various disorders into a single entity that he called dementia praecox, or dementia of early onset, to distinguish this disorder from dementias occurring in old age. He was also the first to describe manic depression (bipolar disorder). Kraepelin divided dementia praecox into three basic subtypes: paranoid, hebephrenic, and catatonic. Kraepelin's system dominated the field of schizophrenia for 30 years. However, it eventually became clear that this disorder was not dementia at all but rather a late-onset mental condition involving psychosis.

In 1911, Swiss psychiatrist Eugen Bleuler[80] convinced the psychiatry world that dementia praecox was an inappropriate term and introduced the term schizophrenia. Bleuler maintained Kraepelin's three subtypes and added a fourth subtype known as schizophrenia simplex. Due to the influence of Freud,[81] Adler,[82] Jung,[83] and others, the treatment of choice for schizophrenia in the early 1900s involved a psychiatrist's couch and exploration of early traumatic experiences, followed by one or more psychodynamic treatment methods. Widespread use of drugs began in the 1950s after the discovery that both Thorazine and Reserpine resulted in great calming and reduction of psychosis in some patients.[76] Over the next two decades, many psychiatrists supplemented their counseling and psychodynamic protocols with powerful psychiatric medications.

Biological Psychiatry

The mid-1960s marked the emergence of *biological psychiatry*, a field that recognized schizophrenia as a medical condition rather than a product of traumatic life experiences.[84] This revolutionary change was influenced by convincing studies of twins[9] proving that schizophrenia ran in families. Table 5-1 shows the increased risk of developing schizophrenia if a blood relative has the disorder.[85] As expected, the highest risk (>50%) is for persons with an identical twin diagnosed with schizophrenia.

Table 5-1. Heritability Risk for Schizophrenia

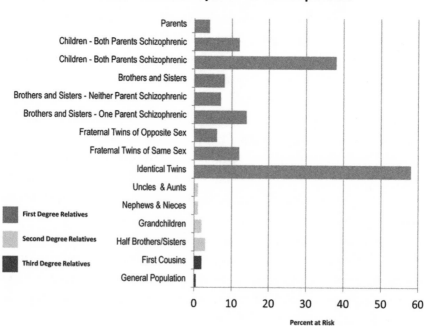

Since the mid-1960s, most schizophrenia patients have left the psychiatrist's couch, and therapy has concentrated on psychiatric medications aimed at correcting brain chemistry and adjusting neurotransmitter activity. Significant benefits were reported for early antipsychotic drugs, including Thorazine, Haldol, Prolixin, Mellaril, Navane, and Stelazine. Unfortunately, each involved a high incidence of serious side effects, including movement disorders, excessive sedation, sleep disorders, weight gain, dry mouth, altered personality, diabetes, and the potentially fatal neuroleptic malignant syndrome. These unpleasant side effects caused many patients to abruptly stop medication (against doctors' orders), usually resulting in dramatic worsening and, in many instances, suicide.

Since the 1990s, second-generation schizophrenia drugs called atypical antipsychotics have been introduced. These medications are generally more effective in combating psychosis and involve reduced side effects. Atypicals are a group of unrelated drugs united by the fact that they work differently from the first-generation antipsychotics. Most of them share the attribute of impacting both serotonin and dopamine receptors. The first atypical antipsychotic was Clozaril, a medication still regarded as highly effective. One potential side effect is a fatal blood disorder requiring frequent lab testing, and many psychiatrists now use Clozaril as a last resort. Popular atypical drugs[86] include Zyprexa, Risperdal, Seroquel, Geodon, Abilify, and Invega, with additional medications under active development.

Use of atypical medications is still a trial-and-error proposition, and the effect of any of these drugs cannot be predicted with confidence. Some patients achieve success with their first atypical, whereas others have tried many atypicals without significant benefit. The good news is that a high percentage of schizophrenia patients can reduce or eliminate troubling psychosis symptoms once they find an atypical that is effective for them. However, most successfully treated patients experience one or more side effects,[87] such as sedation, impaired cognition, socialization deficits, altered personality, movement disorders, diabetes, weight gain, strokes, or neuroleptic malignant syndrome. The atypicals generally offer more effective elimination of psychotic symptoms and somewhat lessened side effects when compared with the first-generation drugs. Another concern has been a 2011 study[88] indicating that atypicals result in gradual shrinkage of the brain's cortex. In summary, atypical antipsychotic medications usually result in impressive benefits, but most patients remain handicapped compared to their pre-breakdown condition, experience serious side effects that may become permanent, and may experience gradual loss of brain cortex volumes.

Schizophrenia Theories

1. *Dopamine theory:* In 1952, Arvid Carlsson[89-90] discovered the neuro-
    transmitter dopamine, which was originally believed to be of little significance.
    However, this belief changed when researchers learned that symptoms of
    paranoid schizophrenia could be produced in normal persons by increasing
    dopamine activity through the use of amphetamines. This led many brain
    researchers to conclude that excessive dopamine activity was the underlying
    cause of schizophrenia. This theory was bolstered by studies that showed
    schizophrenic patients improved after treatment with dopamine-lowering
    medications and worsened when given Ritalin or other amphetamines. The
    dopamine theory was entrenched as the leading explanation of schizophrenia for
    the next 30-40 years, and most of today's medications for this disorder continue
    to be based on this model. This theory can explain psychosis and other positive
    symptoms of schizophrenia, but it cannot explain the cognitive, socialization,
    and other negative symptoms that are classic features of the disorder. In recent
    years, the dopamine theory has lost support due to the emergence of the
    glutamate theory of schizophrenia (see below).

2. *Glutamate theory:* Another explanation for schizophrenia is the glutamate
    theory,[91] which is in harmony with both psychosis symptoms and the
    cognitive deficits seen in many patients. The idea stems from observations that
    phencyclidine hydrochloride (PCP) administered to normal persons can induce
    psychosis that closely resembles schizophrenia.[92] The main action of PCP is
    to reduce glutamate activity at NMDA receptors. This theory received strong
    support when it was learned that increasing NMDA activity (using glycine
    supplements) was effective in reducing schizophrenia symptoms. NMDA
    receptors are unique in that neurotransmission requires simultaneous docking
    of both glutamate and glycine molecules.

    The pharmaceutical industry is actively developing drugs aimed at
    increasing glutamate activity at NMDA receptors. However, the nutrients
    sarcosine, D-serine, and D-cycloserine in early tests have shown promise in
    improving NMDA activity by increasing glycine activity at the synapse.[93]
    When taken together with atypical antipsychotic medications, these nutrients
    have produced reports of improvement in double-blind, placebo-controlled
    testing of schizophrenia patients. Researchers continue to investigate the ability
    of these nutrients to enhance the benefits of medications. However, there is
    also the possibility that these nutrients may produce benefits when used alone,

without the drugs. Early testing indicates that sarcosine is more effective than D-serine or D-cycloserine in the treatment of schizophrenia.

3. *Oxidative stress theory:* There is mounting evidence that excessive oxidative stress in the brain is a distinctive feature of schizophrenia, leading many to believe this may be the primary cause of the disorder.[94-95] Oxidative stress is a condition of excessive production of peroxides and free radicals that results in undesirable chemical reactions (described in Appendix B). Glutathione (GSH) levels are depleted by oxidative free radicals and are low in brains of those with schizophrenia. Moreover, low GSH reduces glutamate activity at NMDA receptors, a condition that can produce hallucinations, delusions, and other classic symptoms of schizophrenia. Recent evidence of neurodegeneration (loss of brain cells) in schizophrenia[96] is consistent with elevated oxidative stress. The many sources of oxidative stress in the brain include heavy metals, viruses, bacteria, injury, inflammation, emotional stress, nuclear radiation, and high iron levels.

    Fortunately, the brain is protected by several antioxidant factors including GSH, metallothionein, selenium, superoxide dismutase (SOD), catalase, vitamin C, and cysteine. The situation may be thought of as a war between the oxidative free radicals and the antioxidant protectors. In schizophrenia, it appears the free radicals have won the war. This could be caused by one of two factors:

    ♦ Excessive environmental insults that produce free radicals
    ♦ Weakened antioxidant protection in the brain

    The strong heritable predisposition for schizophrenia suggests that weak antioxidant protection is the culprit in most cases. The oxidative stress theory of schizophrenia is steadily gaining momentum and may soon achieve equal status with the dopamine and NMDA models.

4. *Epigenetics theory:* Several researchers have proposed that schizophrenia is the result of epigenetic errors that alter expression of genes that impact mental health.[97-98] This concept is supported by the fact that schizophrenia runs in families but does not follow classical Mendelian genetics.[99] For example, there are numerous cases of identical (monozygotic) twins in which only one develops schizophrenia. In addition, decades of research have failed to identify genes responsible for the most common forms of the disease. In contrast, early epigenetics studies have borne fruit. A study of identical twins discordant for

schizophrenia[100] found epigenetic DNA methylation abnormalities in the schizophrenics but not in their twin brothers. In other studies,[101] schizophrenics had higher levels of methylation than depressive controls, resulting in lower gene expression of GAD67, an enzyme that produces the neurotransmitter GABA; the researchers found that methionine worsened symptoms, while valproic acid increased histone acetylation and provided benefits. It seems likely that nutrients that increase acetylation such as folic acid and niacin could provide similar benefits.

As described in Chapter 4, methyl and folate levels can have a powerful epigenetic role in determining which genes are expressed or inhibited. An abnormal methyl/folate ratio can cause altered amounts of important enzymes and transporters needed for proper brain function. Abnormal blood levels of methyl and folate are present in about 70% of all persons diagnosed with schizophrenia. The undermethylation and overmethylation phenotypes of schizophrenia could well be epigenetic in origin. Excessive dopamine activity associated with an elevated methyl/folate ratio involves underproduction of a complex chemical called dopamine active transporter (DAT). This transporter removes dopamine from synapses, sending it back to the original cell for reuse. Overmethylation results in reduced expression of DAT and excessive dopamine activity. This biochemical abnormality is a hallmark of paranoid schizophrenia. In contrast, the epigenetic effect of undermethylation is to reduce activity of serotonin, dopamine, and norepinephrine. In addition, undermethylation appears to influence synaptic NMDA receptor activity and is associated with schizoaffective disorder and delusional disorders. Reduced activity of norepinephrine usually coincides with reduced adrenaline activity that may contribute to catatonic symptoms that are characteristic of schizoaffective disorder and delusional disorder.

The theory that schizophrenia is caused by a virus[102] can be considered a variant of the epigenetic theory, in which a viral insult alters gene expression. The discovery of transgenerational epigenetic inheritance in humans (described in Chapter 4) provides a new explanation for the powerful family heritability of schizophrenia that violates the classic laws of genetics.

If the epigenetics theory turns out to be correct, the impact on schizophrenia prevention and treatment could be massive. Future research might lead to identification of the specific DNA methylation and histone modification errors that produce mental illness—and effective treatments would not be far behind. Epigenetics is an extremely promising area of schizophrenia research that may eventually lead to a cure for this dreaded mental illness.

Biochemical Classification of the Schizophrenias

My analysis of blood and urine testing of 3,600 persons diagnosed with schizophrenia has confirmed Pfeiffer's finding of three distinct chemical classifications or phenotypes

Figure 5-1. Schizophrenia Biotypes

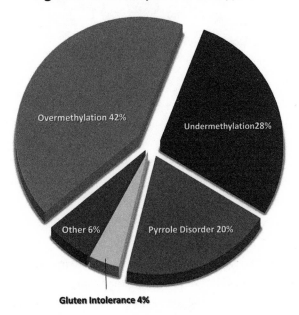

that represent 90% of the cases: overmethylated schizophrenia (42%), undermethylated schizophrenia (28%), and a condition of severe oxidative stress termed pyrrole schizophrenia (20%). Each phenotype involves a distinctive constellation of symptoms and traits that can assist in diagnosis. The primary schizophrenia phenotypes are shown in Figure 5-1. Less common forms of the disease are shown in Figure 5-2.

Differential Diagnosis Factors

Patients who are overmethylated or pyroluric usually exhibit warning signs of the disease before the age of 10, but undermethylated patients may be symptom-free until the breakdown. Chemical analyses of blood and urine provide about 50% of the information required for accurate diagnosis. Symptoms, traits, physical signs, medical history, and family history are equally useful in identifying a patient's schizophrenia biotype. It is often possible to predict a patient's blood and urine chemistry after an in-depth medical history and review of symptoms. Presence (or absence) of key symptoms together with lab chemistries usually enable accurate diagnosis of the schizophrenia biotype.

Figure 5-2. Other Forms of Schizophrenia

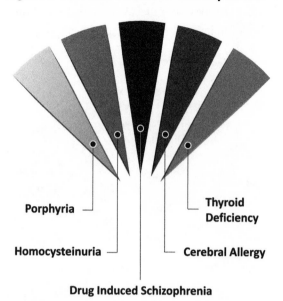

Porphyria

Homocysteinuria

Thyroid
Deficiency

Cerebral Allergy

Drug Induced Schizophrenia

Symptoms during initial breakdown: The striking changes that occur during an initial mental breakdown (prior to psychiatric medications) are especially revealing. Psychiatric medications often mask key symptoms intrinsic to the disease. Behavioral and sensory changes during schizophrenia onset can greatly assist in developing a correct diagnosis:

- Persons who become more physically active and report hearing voices are likely to be overmethylated.
- Patients who shut down with catatonic symptoms usually exhibit undermethylation.
- Schizophrenics who exhibit wild mood swings, great fears, and deteriorate under stress are likely to have pyrrole disorder.

Response to psychiatric medications: This is an area of critical importance that can assist in forming an accurate biochemical diagnosis. Patients and families may give negative ratings for medications that successfully reduced psychosis but that produced unpleasant side effects. The key is to determine if the medication alleviated the psychosis, regardless of side effects. Dramatic worsening of psychiatric symptoms after serotonin-enhancing SSRIs suggests folate insufficiency and methyl overload. Similarly, worsening of psychosis after a benzodiazapine medication suggests a low methyl/folate ratio.

Family history: More than 50% of schizophrenia patients have at least one relative with a serious mental illness. It is very helpful to obtain detailed information about any mentally ill relatives including diagnosis, medication successes and failures, primary symptoms, and behaviors. A more complete list of family history factors is shown in Chapter 10. Identification of relatives with clear indications of a specific biotype can assist the diagnostic process.

Dominance of hallucinations or delusions: The medical evaluation should attempt to determine if the condition is primarily a thought disorder or a sensory disorder. Although there are many exceptions, most patients exhibiting severe delusions are undermethylated, whereas most patients with a dominant symptom of auditory hallucinations are overmethylated. Most pyrrole disorder patients exhibit both delusions and auditory hallucinations.

Psychiatric medication issues: Usually, progress is more rapid and complete if ongoing medication is continued during the first several months of nutrient therapy. We have learned through experience that recovered schizophrenics who completely eliminate psychiatric medication are likely to relapse within a year. As a consequence, we recommend that patients not attempt to cease medication altogether. Many recovered schizophrenics now live quite normal and productive lives while continuing nutrient therapy along with a low dose of an atypical antipsychotic medication. I expect future advances in brain science will provide a roadmap to improved nutrient therapies that will not require a drug medication assist.

After several months of nutrient therapy, some patients report great improvement in psychosis symptoms, anxiety, depression, socialization, and cognition while simultaneously experiencing extreme physical tiredness and reduced energy. I often tell these patients that it's time to celebrate since this means they are getting better—that the nutrient therapy has improved brain function to the extent that ongoing psychiatric medication is now causing excessive sedation. A visit to the psychiatrist will usually result in reduced medication dosage and a return to normal energy.

Recovery timeline: It is very important that families be informed of the expected recovery timeline so that they not become unduly discouraged by lack of early progress.

- Mentally ill patients with pyrrole disorder usually improve significantly during the first two to four weeks of nutrient therapy, with progress continuing for two to four months.

◆ Most overmethylated psychotics are greatly troubled during the first three weeks of treatment, with clear improvement beginning during week four.

◆ Delusional undermethylated patients usually report little or no progress over the first four to six weeks and then experience a gradual recovery during the next six months. Many of these patients report a return to a normal life.

Overmethylation Biotype of Schizophrenia

Overmethylation is the dominant chemical imbalance for about 42% of persons diagnosed with schizophrenia. Laboratory indications include whole blood histamine levels below 40 ng/ml, absolute basophil levels below 30, and serum copper higher than 120 mcg/dl. This schizophrenia phenotype involves excessive activity at dopamine and

---

Table 5-2.
Symptoms and Traits – Overmethylated Schizophrenia

-- Auditory hallucinations	-- Paranoia
-- High anxiety and panic tendency	-- Depression
-- Hyperactivity	-- Sleep disorder
-- Low libido	-- Tinnitus
-- Religiosity	-- Upper body/neck/head pain
-- Low blood histamine	-- Hirsutism
-- Low absolute basophils	-- Food/chemical sensitivities
-- Tendency to be overweight	-- Artistic or musical ability
-- Nervous legs, pacing	-- Copper overload
-- Postpartum onset of psychosis	-- Estrogen intolerance
-- Adverse reaction to SSRIs	-- Antihistamine intolerance
-- Adverse reaction to methionine	-- Adverse reaction to SAMe
-- Improvement after benzodiazepines	-- Improvement after lithium
-- Dry eyes and mouth	-- History of eczema
-- Belief that everyone thinks ill of them	-- Self-mutilation
-- Low motivation during school years	-- Obsessions
-- High pain threshold	-- Absence of seasonal allergies
-- Diagnosis of paranoid schizophrenia	-- Frenetic activity

norepinephrine receptors, possibly caused by epigenetic inhibition of dopamine active transporters (DATs) and norepinephrine transporters (NETs) and elevated copper levels. Primary symptoms usually include auditory hallucinations, paranoia, agitation, and extreme anxiety. The most common diagnosis is paranoid schizophrenia.

Table 5-2 presents a list of symptoms and traits associated with this disorder. It's important to note that many of these symptoms may be absent for individual patients and that presence of 30-50% of the factors is a positive indication of overmethylation. The most significant symptoms of overmethylated schizophrenia are auditory hallucinations, severe anxiety, high physical activity, and paranoia.

Case Histories

The following case histories summarize treatment of the overmethylation phenotype of schizophrenia. They are *not* presented as evidence of treatment effectiveness; they are provided to illustrate the clinical approach.

Schizoprenia Case History 1 – Overmethylation

Judy W., age 26, was working as a nurse when she developed a sleep disorder followed by high anxiety, a collapse in work performance, and auditory hallucinations. She reported a persistent condemning male voice telling her she was worthless and should kill herself. Judy received a leave of absence and returned home, but her illness progressively worsened. She saw a psychiatrist and experienced weekly counseling and group therapy that didn't bear fruit. She was hospitalized for a week and began taking Zyprexa, Tegretol, and Zoloft, which reduced the hallucinations and allowed her to sleep.

Judy's maternal grandmother had a history of severe anxiety and depression. As a child, Judy underachieved in school but had many friends. She especially loved art and music. Metabolic testing revealed a very depressed blood histamine level of 10 ng/ml, and she was diagnosed with overmethylation. In addition, she exhibited elevated copper and depressed zinc levels. Judy was treated with folic acid, zinc, niacin and vitamins B-6, B-12, C, and E, which she took along with her medication. Her nutrient therapy was aimed at reducing norepinephrine and dopamine levels while increasing GABA. She reported a worsening of anxiety the first three weeks, followed by clear improvement during month two. Within six months, her symptoms had nearly disappeared and she returned to work after a year's absence. Her psychiatrist has weaned her from Tegrerol and Zoloft, and she continues on a low dose of Zyprexa.

Schizoprenia Case History 2 – Overmethylation

Robert, age 25, sought nutrient therapy after several unsuccessful trials of counseling and psychiatric medication. He was employed as an air traffic controller in a southern state but had experienced auditory hallucinations and high anxiety for the past year. He was quite paranoid and secretive and was afraid of losing his job. He complained of occasional uncertainty whether a voice was that of a pilot or was a hallucination.

There was no known history of mental illness in the family. He complained of food and chemical sensitivities and had received allergy treatments as a child. He had been very sociable prior to his psychosis symptoms but had become a loner. He exhibited several overmethylation symptoms including difficulty sleeping, low libido, nervous legs, and ringing in the ears (tinnitus). He had a heavy beard, and his chest was covered with thick black hair. Robert's testing indicated overmethylation (depressed blood histamine of 26 ng/ml), and he was placed on a regimen of folic acid, vitamins B-3, B-6, B-12, C, and E together with supplements of zinc, manganese, and chromium. At his annual follow-up visit, Robert reported that the voices had disappeared and he felt in good health. He faithfully returns for biochemical testing once yearly.

Undermethylation Biotype of Schizophrenia

Severely depressed methyl/folate ratio is present in about 28% of the schizophrenia population. The dominant symptom is usually delusions, although mild hallucinations are sometimes present. Laboratory indications are whole blood histamine above 70 ng/ml, elevated blood basophils, and depressed SAMe/SAH ratio. Most undermethylated persons in the general population are high achievers in good mental health. However, most mentally ill persons exhibiting this imbalance respond to methylation therapies. This form of schizophrenia involves low activity of serotonin, dopamine, and norepinephrine, possibly caused by epigenetic overexpression of SERT (serotonin transporter), DAT, and NET transporters at synapses. Low glutamate activity at NMDA receptors is also suspected. Typical symptoms include delusions, OCD behaviors, high internal anxiety, and catatonic tendencies.

Table 5-3 presents distinctive symptoms and traits associated with the undermethylated biotype of schizophrenia. The presence of 30-50% of the factors may be sufficient for diagnosis. Many of these patients have a prior diagnosis of

Table 5-3.
Symptoms and Traits – Undermethylated Schizophrenia

-- Severe delusions

-- History of perfectionism

-- Seasonal inhalant allergies

-- Very high libido

-- Diagnosis of delusional disorder

-- Good response to antihistamines

-- High fluidity (tears, saliva, etc.)

-- Good response to SSRIs

-- High accomplishment before onset

-- Adverse reaction to folic acid

-- Sparse chest/leg/arm hair

-- Suicidal tendencies

-- Addictiveness

-- Phobias

-- Infrequent and terse speech

-- Peptic ulcers

-- Denial of illness

-- Noncompliance with therapies

-- Belief that CIA or FBI is after them

-- Attempt to hide the illness

-- Vegetarian diet

-- Obsessive/compulsive tendencies

-- Self-motivated during school years

-- Dietary inflexibility

-- Diagnosis of schizoaffective disorder

-- Adverse reaction to benzodiazepines

-- Low tolerance for pain

-- Catatonic behavior during illness onset

-- Very strong-willed

-- Slenderness

-- History of competitiveness in sports

-- Large nose and ears

-- Prior diagnosis of OCD or ODD

-- Ritualistic behaviors

-- Calm demeanor but high inner tension

-- Frequent headaches

-- Family history of high accomplishment

-- Blankminded appearance

-- Poor concentration endurance

-- Social isolation

-- Belief that a friend or relative is an alien

-- Rumination about past events

schizoaffective disorder or delusional disorder. Common symptoms include belief that the CIA or FBI is following them, that their parents are aliens, or that a satellite in outer space is beaming painful rays into their brain. Most undermethylated schizophrenics have ritualistic behaviors and strong obsessive-compulsive tendencies. They may have extreme inner anxiety that is hidden behind a calm exterior. Ususally the delusional beliefs are unshakable, and the patient will refuse to consider the possibility that he/she is in error. The following case histories illustrate the undermethylation phenotype of schizophrenia.

Schizoprenia Case History 3 – Undermethylation

David was a brilliant 22-year-old PhD candidate at Berkeley who developed disturbing symptoms after breaking up with his girlfriend. He stopped attending classes, told friends that Russian agents were trying to kill him, and would sit for hours with a blank expression. He was diagnosed with schizoaffective disorder, hospitalized for 10 days, and medicated with Zyprexa, Depakote, and Zoloft. Despite significant improvement, David was unable to resume his studies or hold a job. He reported a 50 pound weight gain and had isolated himself from his friends.

A biochemical evaluation revealed symptoms of undermethylation, including a history of seasonal allergies, perfectionism, competitiveness in sports, and sparse chest hair. His blood histamine level was extremely elevated at 170 ng/ml, and he was treated with SAMe, methionine, calcium, magnesium, zinc, serine, and vitamins A, B-6, C, D, and E. His family reported no change for six weeks, followed by slow improvement. After a year of nutrient therapy, David reported a nearly complete recovery, and his psychiatrist weaned him from Depakote and Zoloft and reduced the dosage of Zyprexa. He has held a job as a computer specialist for the past five years and is now married and starting a family. He continues to comply with his nutrient program and a low dosage of Zyprexa and reports an absence of side effects.

Schizophrenia Case History 4 – Undermethylation

George dropped out of high school and found work at an auto assembly plant in Michigan. He experienced a mental breakdown after his 21st birthday and was fired from his job. George was diagnosed with paranoid schizophrenia, the same condition that had afflicted his mother. He was evaluated by a psychiatrist but refused to comply with medication.

After four hospitalizations, George agreed to undergo biochemical testing. He arrived for his first appointment wearing a metal helmet and had heavy chains wrapped around his neck. George explained that the metal was necessary to keep him from floating up into outer space where he would die. He also believed that his parents were aliens and not the people he lived with as a child. His evaluation revealed several undermethylation symptoms including hayfever, high libido, excessive saliva and tears, sparse chest hair, and chain smoking. His blood histamine and absolute basophil levels were both elevated, and he was treated with methionine, calcium, magnesium, zinc, chromium, and vitamins A, B-6, C, D, and E. In addition he was given the nutrient inositol to help with sleep. George had chronic problems with compliance, but he reported significant improvement after six months.

At a follow-up visit, he no longer was weighted down with metal and agreed to see a psychiatrist and receive low-dose medication support. After several years of wellness, he stopped compliance with his medication and nutrients, and his delusions returned within a few months. He has since been compliant with treatment and reports that he is doing well.

Pyrrole Disorder Biotype of Schizophrenia

This phenotype involves a severe overload of oxidative stress that impairs brain function. This condition usually results in very elevated levels of pyrroles in urine along with severe deficiencies of zinc and vitamin B-6. These chemical imbalances were originally attributed to deviant biochemical processes in bone marrow and spleen, but there are other sources of oxidative stress that also elevate pyrroles.

Most persons with elevated pyrroles have mild symptoms that do not interfere with daily living. However, about 20% of schizophrenics exhibit a severe version of this imbalance and report improvement following aggressive therapy with zinc and vitamin B-6. This condition involves free-radical oxidative stress and depleted levels of glutathione, metallothionein, and other protective proteins causing inhibition of glutamate activity at NMDA receptors. Primary symptoms of pyrrole disorder generally include the following:

- Extreme mood swings
- Sensitivity to light and noise
- Poor stress control
- Severe anxiety
- Little or no dream recall
- Preference for spicy foods
- Abnormal fat distribution

A study of 67 schizophrenics found that pyrolurics were very deficient in arachidonic acid, an omega-6 fatty acid. This may explain the symptoms of dry skin and abnormal fat distribution associated with this disorder. Many pyroluric schizophrenics report benefits from supplements of primrose oil, a source of omega-6. Non-pyrrole schizophrenia phenotypes generally exhibit low omega-3 levels and omega-6 overload. A recent study[27] reported biotin deficiency in pyrrole patients.

Most pyroluric schizophrenics report symptoms of zinc and vitamin B-6 deficiency from early childhood. Physical symptoms include delayed growth, poor

---

Table 5-4.
Symptoms and Traits – Pyrrole Schizophrenia

-- Poor stress control	-- Severe oxidative stress
-- Elevated kryptopyrroles in urine	-- Poor short-term memory
-- Sensitivity to bright lights	-- Sensitivity to loud noises
-- Morning nausea	-- Affinity for spicy and salty foods
-- Tendency to delay or skip breakfast	-- Abnormal fat distribution
-- Very dry skin	-- Delicate facial features
-- Pale skin, inability to tan	-- Extreme mood swings
-- High irritability and temper	-- History of a reading disorder
-- History of underachievement	-- Severe inner tension
-- Little or no dream recall	-- Frequent infections
-- Autoimmune disorders	-- Premature graying of hair
-- White spots on fingernails	-- Abnormal menstrual periods
-- Poor growth	-- Poor muscle development
-- Coarse eyebrow hair	-- "Fruity" breath and/or body odor
-- Stretch marks (striae) on skin	-- Spleen area pain
-- Severe depression	-- Severe anxiety
-- Fear of airplane travel, tornadoes, etc	-- Histrionic behavior
-- Obsessions with negative thoughts	-- Joint pains
-- Delayed puberty	-- Poor wound healing
-- Dark or mauve-colored urine	-- Psoriasis
-- Abnormal EEG	-- Tendency to stay up very late

wound healing, dry skin, white spots on fingernails, delayed puberty, acne, and inability to tan. Most pyrolurics have a history of academic underachievement that has been attributed to severe vitamin B-6 deficiency that can impair short-term memory. Mood swings may occur many times daily, and a common diagnosis is rapid-cycling bipolar disorder. The onset usually occurs during a period of extreme stress. Schizophrenics with this imbalance may have a combination of delusions and auditory hallucinations. They live in a world of fear and do not attempt to hide their anxieties. Many are prone to impulsive actions that may be very dangerous. High doses of tranquilizing medications are often employed to combat wild behavior. The primary symptoms and traits associated with the pyrrole phenotype of schizophrenia are presented in Table 5-4.

The following case history illustrates the evaluation and treatment approach for a schizophrenic patient diagnosed with severe pyrrole disorder.

Schizophrenia Case History 5 – Pyrrole Disorder

Mary became the head of a successful family business in Wisconsin at age 29. Three years later, she suffered a severe mental breakdown when her mother was killed in an automobile accident. After many unsuccessful medication trials, she became suicidal with daily episodes of hysteria. A biochemical evaluation revealed several classic symptoms of pyrrole disorder, including morning nausea, aversion to sunlight, absence of dream recall, history of severe sunburn, preference for spicy Mexican and Indian foods, and abnormal menstrual cycles. She also exhibited the classic pyroluric fat distribution, with a slender neck and thin wrists and ankles along with huge amounts of fat at her midsection and upper thighs. Mary's lab testing showed a single abnormality: a urine pyrrole level exceeding 150 µg/ml, more than 10 times the normal level. Her nutrient therapy involved very high doses of zinc and vitamin B-6 together with augmenting nutrients. She responded quickly, and the family reported great improvement after 30 days. She returned for a follow-up evaluation in three months and appeared to be completely recovered, despite the absence of psychiatric medication. Mary resumed her role as the leader of the family business, but she suffered two serious relapses in subsequent years when she temporarily stopped the nutrient program. Mary's family reports she has been well for the past six years, and the family business is prospering.

Low-Incidence Biotypes

As described in the previous section, about 90% of schizophrenics exhibit overmethylation, undermethylation, or pyrrole disorder as their dominant chemical imbalance. Gluten intolerance appears to be responsible for an additional 4% of persons diagnosed with schizophrenia. The remaining 6% involve a collection of relatively rare mental illness biotypes,[28-29] including thyroid deficiency, polydipsia, homocysteinuria, drug-induced psychosis, and porphyria. An efficient clinical approach is to determine the presence (or absence) of the three major biotypes while being alert for indications of gluten intolerance or thyroid deficiency. If all of these conditions are ruled out, the rarer biotypes should be investigated.

Gluten intolerance: Many cases of childhood schizophrenia can be traced to celiac disease that involves intolerance to gluten grains. This disorder can also occur in young adults, most commonly in the third decade of life. This condition is associated with incomplete breakdown of gluten proteins in the GI tract, resulting in small proteins called gluteomorphins that can pass into the bloodstream and access the brain. The net result can be brain inflammation and disturbed function of brain receptors. Early symptoms include bloating, excessive gas, and explosive bowel movements. This condition can be effectively treated by strict elimination of wheat, rye, and some other cereal grains from the diet. A family history of gluten intolerance, Crohn's disease, colitis, or other malabsorptive disease is a warning sign of this disorder. Thousands of persons have tragically suffered a lifetime of severe mental illness that could have been completely overcome by a special diet.

Thyroid deficiency: Dr. Pfeiffer reported that about 1 case of schizophrenia in 200 resulted from severe thyroid deficiency and that standard treatment with either Synthroid or Armour thyroid often resulted in complete recovery. He found that laboratory thyroid panels often failed to detect thyroid deficiency and recommended a thyroid trial for patients exhibiting symptoms of this disorder such as low body temperature, cold extremities, dry skin, hair loss, and low energy.

Polydipsia: Excessive drinking of water can result in psychosis and a diagnosis of schizophrenia. I once met a successful businessman who was diagnosed with schizophrenia at the age of 57, with no prior history of mental problems. His illness began with a sleep medication that resulted in dry mouth and constant thirst. His condition gradually deteriorated, and within a year, he was experiencing anxiety, depression, auditory hallucinations, and delusional beliefs. He had had spent several months in a mental hospital and was taking 14 separate medications daily. His lab results included very low serum sodium and potassium levels, and his urine had a water-like specific gravity of 1.000 with very low creatinine levels. He estimated his water intake at four gallons daily. Treatment simply involved discontinuation of the sleep medication and restricting water intake. Within six weeks, he reported a complete recovery and was able to eliminate all of the medications. His sleep disorder returned and was resolved with supplements of the nutrient inositol.

Homocysteinuria: This rare metabolic disorder can produce symptoms that are indistinguishable from schizophrenia. The usual cause is a genetic lack of an enzyme needed to control levels of the amino acid homocysteine. Most cases can be traced to deficiency of the cystathionine β-synthase (CBS) enzyme (converts homocysteine and serine to cytathionine) or the methylenetetrahydrofolate reductase (MTHFR) enzyme (converts homocysteine to methionine). Dysfunction in these enzymes causes impairment to the methylation cycle (described in Appendix A) and reduced production of glutathione and other antioxidants. This condition can be treated with supplements of vitamins B-6 and B-12 in conjunction with folic acid, serine, and trimethylglycine (TMG). This biotype represents less than 0.1% of the schizophrenia population. Early diagnosis and detection are essential since this disorder is associated with progressive mental retardation and is also associated with cardiovascular diseases.

Drug-induced schizophrenia: There are dozens of psychiatric drugs that can produce full-blown symptoms of schizophrenia in certain persons. It is important to determine if the onset of mental illness occurred soon after starting a medication. I've encountered occasional patients diagnosed with paranoid schizophrenia who were faithfully continuing a medication that had caused their illness. In these cases, complete recovery may result from simply weaning the patient from the medication. I've met other heavily sedated patients who were unnecessarily taking an atypical antipsychotic drug after a single psychotic episode that apparently was caused by a suspect medication or recreational drug.

Illegal drugs of abuse including cocaine, LSD, PCP, and amphetamines can produce a side effect of psychosis in highly sensitive persons. In rare occasions, a psychosis condition can be solely the result of continuing drug abuse. Most drug abusers deny their use of illegal drugs, and this condition can be very difficult to diagnose. Urine testing for illegal drugs is very inefficient, but a radioimmunoassay of hair (RIAH) test can determine the nature and frequency of drug abuse.

Most patients with drug-induced schizophrenia that persists after abstinence exhibit the undermethyation biotype.

The porphyrias: Porphyrias[103] are a group of inherited or acquired disorders of certain enzymes in the heme biosynthetic pathway. Typical symptoms include abdominal pain, hallucinations, depression, paranoia, and anxiety. Diagnosis is complicated by the existence of eight different genetic forms of porphyria that have symptom variations. In my experience, coproporphyria is the most common type of porphyria inappropriately diagnosed as schizophrenia. Porphyrin molecules contain rings of pyrrole groups, and severe elevations of urine pyrroles and toxic metals are usually present along with a pronounced lack of zinc and vitamin B-6. Despite the presence of these correctable chemical imbalances, nutrient therapy has generally resulted in disappointingly minor improvements in these patients. More research is needed to achieve a better understanding of the biochemistry of the porphyrias.

The Walsh Theory of Schizophrenia

A flaw in existing theories has been the failure to recognize that schizophrenia is an umbrella term used for a variety of psychotic disorders, each presenting a distinctive set of symptoms and traits. It seems very unlikely that these disparate mental illnesses (a) arise from the same underlying cause, (b) share the same neurotransmission abnormalities, and (c) are best served by the same treatment approach. I believe a proper theory of schizophrenia must include the following elements:

- Separate causation for the major phenotypes
- Explanation for the mental breakdown event that usually occurs in late adolescence or young adulthood
- Explanation for the lifelong persistence of schizophrenia after the mental breakdown
- Explanation of why this familial (heritable) disorder violates classical laws of Mendelian genetics

After working with more than 3,000 patients diagnosed with schizophrenia, I eventually discovered that the vast majority shared two important characteristics: (1) vulnerability to epigenetic errors that can alter gene expression and (2) weakened protection against oxidative stress. These insights led to my theory of schizophrenia which is presented below.

Thesis 1: Predisposition to schizophrenia involves fetal programming errors that cause lifelong vulnerability to oxidative stresses. These programming errors can result from a variety of causes including the following: (a) an abnormal in utero methylation environment, (b) exposure to environmental toxins, (c) genetic weakness in oxidative protection, and (d) medication side effects.

Thesis 2: The mental breakdown event is triggered by overwhelming oxidative stress that alters DNA and histone marks that regulate gene expression. Cancer research has provided examples of cumulative oxidative stresses that eventually alter gene marks, producing an enduring disease condition. The onset of schizophrenia occurs when oxidative stresses exceed the threshold level needed to alter chromatin marks that control gene expression.

Thesis 3: Epigenetic changes are responsible for continuing psychotic tendencies after the breakdown event. A psychotic breakdown is usually followed by a lifetime of mental illness and misery, despite intensive therapies. This often permanent change in functioning results from altered DNA or histone marks that regulate gene expression. Since the deviant marks are maintained during future cell divisions, the condition doesn't go away.

Thesis 4: The three major phenotypes of schizophrenia develop in individuals who exhibit overmethylation, undermethyation, or overwhelming oxidative stress:

A. <u>Overmethylation</u>: About 42% of persons diagnosed with schizophrenia exhibit severe overmethylation together with oxidative overload. Mental breakdowns generally occur during severe physical or emotional traumatic events that sharply increase oxidative stress and produce deviant gene marks. This schizophrenia biotype is a sensory disorder that generally involves auditory, tactile, or visual hallucinations. This condition is associated with elevated activity of dopamine and norepinephrine and reduced glutamate activity at NMDA receptors. The most common DSM-IV-TR diagnosis is paranoid schizophrenia.

B. <u>Undermethylation</u>: About 28% of persons diagnosed with schizophrenia exhibit undermethylation together with weak antioxidant protection. Mental breakdowns generally occur during severe physical or emotional traumatic events that produce a separate set of altered gene marks. This schizophrenia biotype essentially is a thought disorder with delusions and catatonic tendencies as the primary symptoms. This condition is associated with low activity at serotonin, dopamine, and NMDA receptors. The most common DSM-IV-TR diagnoses are schizoaffective disorder or delusional disorder.

C. Severe oxidative overload: The third major schizophrenia phenotype develops in persons with an inborn severe deficit in antioxidant protection. This condition is arbitrarily termed pyrrole disorder due to the presence of excessive pyrrole levels in blood and urine. Mental breakdowns occur for these persons during periods of extreme physical or mental stress in which deviant epigenetic marks are established. This condition is characterized by extraordinary anxiety and rapid mood swings, and it often involves both auditory hallucinations and delusional beliefs. Brain chemistry abnormalities include (a) depressed glutamate activity at NMDA receptors and (b) very depressed GABA activity.

Thesis 5: Failure to follow classical laws of genetic inheritance results from the epigenetic nature of schizophrenia. Schizophrenia is strongly heritable (runs in families) but fails to obey Mendel's classic laws of genetic inheritance. There are countless examples of identical twins where one sibling develops the disorder and the other does not. In addition, intensive research efforts to identify the schizophrenia gene (or genes) have met with little success. Epigenetics provides two explanations for the non-Mendelian nature of schizophrenia: (a) environmental insults are required to produce deviant epigenetic marks, and environmental conditions are highly variable for different individuals, and (b) transgenerational epigenetic inheritance contributes to schizophrenia heritability by transmitting deviant epigenetic marks to one's children and grandchildren.

CHAPTER 6

DEPRESSION

Introduction

Depression is the most prevalent of mental disorders and results in health care costs of billions of dollars annually. Depression exists in all cultures and ethnic groups throughout the world. It strikes about one-sixth of all Americans, but only about 50% of those persons seek medical treatment. Typical symptoms include chronic sadness, feelings of worthlessness or guilt, social withdrawal, agitation, problems with concentration, and difficulty sleeping. Depression is a broad term used to describe a variety of medical conditions,[73] including dysthymia, bipolar disorder, cyclothymic disorder, substance-induced mood disorder, seasonal affective disorder, and postpartum depression. Depression can result in a lifetime of misery and is believed responsible for about 60% of suicides in the USA.

Historical Perspective

References to depression are found in earliest recorded history. Hindu sacred writings (*Vedas*) dating back to 1,500 BC emphasized the prevention of mental pain. The Old Testament describes King Saul's severe depression and ultimate suicide. Ancient civilizations thought depression was caused by evil spirits that could be released by drilling holes in the skull. In 440 BC, Hippocrates dismissed this belief and insisted that depression must be explained by natural causes such as the flow of bile to the brain. The term melancholia derived from the Greek word for black bile. In the next century, Plato erroneously revived the theory that depression was caused by mystical forces, but Aristotle later rejected this belief. The Roman philosopher Cicero theorized that depression resulted from life experiences and advocated a treatment similar to counseling.

Very little progress was made in the understanding or treatment of depression over the next 1,700 years. Real progress began in the 19th century when depression was recognized as a medical condition, and the medical and scientific communities actively sought effective therapies. The term depression (from the latin verb *deprimere*, to press down) soon became synonymous with melancholia. Throughout the early

1900s, the predominant belief was that depression resulted from flawed or traumatic life experiences. Meyer, Freud, Adler, Jung, and others developed talk therapies and counseling techniques aimed at (a) identifying the events or conditions that caused the depression and (b) treating the condition.

In the mid-20th century, some researchers theorized that depression was caused by chemical imbalances in the brain,[104] based on observations that Reserpine and Isoniazid medications altered neurotransmitter levels and affected depressive symptoms. This gave birth to the field of biological psychiatry and revolutionary approaches for treating depression.[105] Within a few years, a monoamine theory of depression was generally accepted by the psychiatry community.[106] This theory asserted that clinical depression was caused by low synaptic activities of serotonin and norepinephrine in the brain. Since 1975, the lion's share of psychiatry research has been aimed at developing medications that improve brain function. Tricyclic amines and monoamine oxidase inhibitors were widely used depression medications in the 1980s but have been largely replaced by SSRIs since 1987. Prozac, Paxil, Zoloft, and other SSRIs have benefitted millions of depression patients, but nagging problems with unpleasant side effects remain.

As introduced in Chapter 4, common side effects of SSRIs include loss of libido, weight gain, clinical worsening, increased suicide risk, agitation, hostility, anxiety, insomnia, and weight loss.[107] Some depressed patients benefit from a specific SSRI without significant side effects, but others may become worse using the same medication. For some persons, switching to another SSRI can be successful. The pharmaceutical industry continues to devote massive research funds aimed at developing improved antidepressant medications.

Biochemical Classification of Depression

In 1978, inspired by Carl Pfeiffer's success in the classification of schizophrenia, I began collecting laboratory chemistries for persons diagnosed with clinical depression. After 20 years, the database amounted to more than 300,000 chemical analyses of blood and urine for 2,800 depressed persons. Examination of this data revealed that this depressed population was biochemically different from the general population. The database also contained detailed information for factors such as symptoms, traits, medical history, allergies, and responses to medications. Eventually, I discovered that the depressive population could be separated into the five major chemical classifications or biotypes shown in Figure 6-1.

In addition to unique biochemistry, each of the five depression biotypes exhibited a high incidence of distinctive symptoms, traits, and physical characteristics. Based on biochemistry, symptoms, response to psychiatric medications, etc., neurotransmitter

Figure 6-1. Depression Biotypes

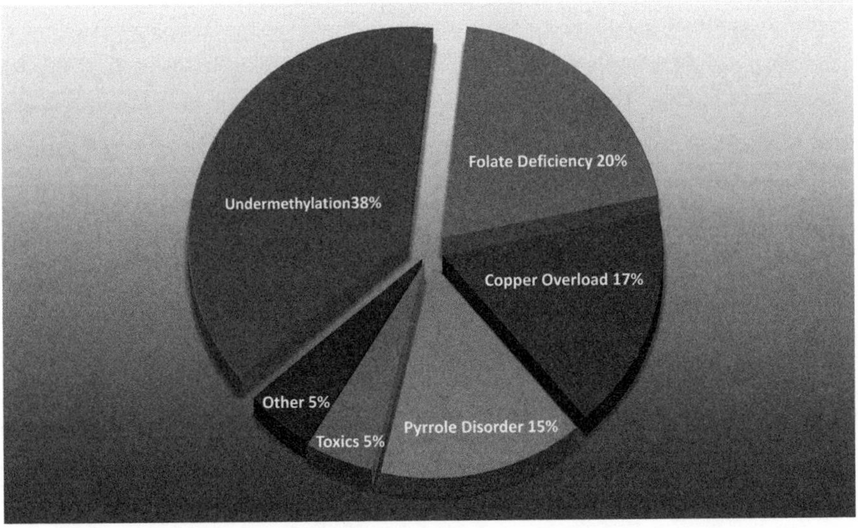

tendencies have been identified for the major biotypes as shown in Table 6-1.

Most depressives in the undermethylation biotype exhibit classic symptoms of low serotonin and report improved moods after serotonin-enhancing SSRI medications. In contrast, the folate deficiency biotype is associated with elevated serotonin and dopamine activity and intolerance to SSRI medications. High-copper depressives have a strong tendency for reduced dopamine and elevated norepinephrine activity. Persons in the pyrrole biotype experience a nasty double deficiency of serotonin and GABA, which is the chief inhibitory (calming) neurotransmitter in the central

Table 6-1.
Depression Biotypes and Neurotransmitter Imbalances

Depression Biotype	Neurotransmitter Activity
Undermethylation	Reduced serotonin, dopamine
Folate deficiency	Elevated serotonin, dopamine
Copper overload	Elevated norepinephrine
Pyrrole disorder	Reduced serotonin, GABA

nervous system. A serious toxic metal overload can impair the blood-brain barrier, disable key antioxidant proteins in the brain, damage the myelin sheath, and alter the concentrations of certain neurotransmitters.

Separate nutrient therapy protocols have been developed for each of the five depression biotypes. These therapies are designed to normalize key chemical factors that influence neurotransmitter synthesis and synaptic activity. Many common psychiatric illnesses involve inherited imbalances of specific minerals, vitamins, and amino acids that can alter neurotransmitter activity in the brain. Individualized nutrient therapy is an effective clinical approach for correcting these chemical imbalances and benefitting patients with depression.

Undermethylated Depression

Approximately 38% of individuals in my depression database exhibit undermethylation as their dominant chemical imbalance. These persons appear to be highly sensitive to the methyl/folate ratio in the brain. They thrive on SAMe, methionine, and other powerful methylating agents but are strikingly intolerant to folates that also promote methylation. As described in Chapter 4, methyl and folate have opposite epigenetic effects on expression of transporters that control synaptic activity of serotonin, dopamine, and norepinephrine. An abnormally low methyl/folate ratio is associated with low serotonin, dopamine, and norepinephrine activity at brain synapses. Most undermethylated depressives exhibit classic symptoms of low serotonin and report lessening of depression symptoms after taking serotonin-enhancing SSRI medications. Table 6-2 presents a partial list of symptoms and traits associated with this depression biotype.

Diagnosis of undermethylated depression is based on blood and urine chemistries along with evaluation of the symptoms and traits shown in Table 6-2. Important indicators of this syndrome include a whole blood histamine level above 70 ng/ml and a depressed SAMe/SAH ratio in combination with key symptoms and traits such as OCD tendencies, seasonal allergies, and a history of pefectionism. Methylation therapy for low-serotonin depressives is unique because of the need to limit folate intake that would increase production of SERT and reduce serotonin activity. The nutrient factor with the greatest positive impact for treatment of this depression biotype is direct methylation, either in the form of SAMe or the amino acid methionine.

Folate, choline, DMAE, and pantothenic acid supplements must be avoided since they increase chromatin acetylation and SERT levels. A high percentage of these patients exhibit low stores of calcium, vitamin D, and magnesium and thrive

Table 6-2.
Symptoms and Traits – Undermethylated Depression

-- Good response to SSRIs	-- Good response to SAMe, methionine
-- Adverse reaction to folic acid	-- High inner tension
-- Obsessive-compulsive tendencies	-- History of perfectionism
-- Self-motivated	-- Seasonal inhalant allergies
-- Good response to antihistamines	-- High libido
-- Low tolerance for pain	-- High fluidity (tears, saliva, etc.)
-- Very strong-willed	-- Competitiveness in sports
-- High suicidal tendency	-- Addictiveness
-- Sparse chest/leg/arm hair	-- Calm demeanor
-- Denial of depression	-- Frequent headaches
-- Family history of high accomplishment	-- Noncompliance with therapies
-- Rumination about past events	-- Oppositional defiance as child

on supplements of these nutrients. In addition, nutrients that enhance synthesis of serotonin can be helpful (e.g., tryptophan, vitamin B-6, 5-HTP). Augmenting nutrients include vitamins A, C, and E.

Most undermethylated depressives exhibit low levels of homocysteine, but others may exhibit elevated levels of this well-known cardiovascular risk factor. Since methylation therapy tends to elevate this biochemical, some patients must have treatment to normalize homocysteine levels prior to use of SAMe or methionine. In most cases, supplementation with serine and vitamin B-6 for a few weeks can bring homocysteine down to a safe level. Experience with hundreds of undermethylated depressives has confirmed that folates, choline, manganese, copper, and DMAE tend to worsen their depression and must be strictly avoided.

Depression Case History 1 – Undermethylation
Charles, age 52, was a successful executive in the steel industry and father of six children. Despite impressive career and financial successes, he had been depressed for more than 15 years with persistent thoughts of suicide.

He reported that depression didn't affect his work performance but was causing problems in his second marriage. Charles described himself as a driven perfectionist who loved competitive sports. Symptoms of undermethylation included hay fever, high libido, internal anxiety, frequent headaches, and sparse hair on his chest, arms, and legs. Charles reported that Prozac, Zoloft, and Paxil all lessened depression, but side effects including a loss of sex drive, nausea, and a worsening of the headaches caused him to stop these medications. His lab work revealed an extreme elevation of blood histamine (142 ng/ml), a mild elevation of urine pyrroles, and low-normal homocysteine. His treatment consisted of SAMe, methionine, zinc, serine, calcium, magnesium, and vitamins A, B-6, C, D, and E. Charles complained of a lack of progress after two months of treatment, but he reported improvement during month 3. After 12 months of treatment, he returned for testing and stated that his depression had been nearly gone for several months. He complained that compliance was difficult and was prescribed a compounded program that reduced the number of capsules. We have not received reports of returning depression since that time.

Depression Case History 2 – Undermethylation

Julie, age 42, had been married and divorced three times and was living with a new boyfriend and her four children in Wisconsin. At age 16, she was diagnosed with oppositional-defiant disorder. She reported intermittent depression since her first marriage at age 19. She said her school grades were excellent until high school when she became more interested in boys than academics. She dropped out of college during her freshman year to marry an older man. Since that time, she experienced episodes of chronic depression, especially in late spring and early fall. She had worked as a hair stylist and a waitress, and she was presently a sales clerk in a large department store. She reported several symptoms of undermethylated depression, including a shopping disorder, habitual cigarette smoking, sensitivity to ragweed and grasses, and a good response to antihistamines. Julie had tried three separate antidepressants but claimed none were effective. The primary laboratory finding was an elevated blood histamine level of 82 ng/ml. Julie had limited funds and decided she couldn't afford to take SAMe, a relatively expensive supplement. Her treatment involved high dosages of methionine, calcium, and magnesium together with zinc, vitamins B-6, C, D, and E, and chromium. Julie returned for a follow-up evaluation after 6 months and reported that her depression was gone but that she still had problems with allergies and shopping binges. She expressed satisfaction with the treatment results and said her boyfriend had decided to marry her since she "had become a nicer person."

Many persons suffering from undermethyated depression have two traits that make successful treatment difficult. First of all, they have an innate tendency for noncompliance with any medical treatment. Some admit they won't take aspirin during a headache, even though they know it would help them. The second trait is a tendency to deny depression, even when the problem is severe. An example of this involves a retired judge from Maryland whom I met during his initial clinical visit. His wife sought me out with a plea to help her husband who had terrible depression that greatly concerned her. I met privately with the judge who laughed and convincingly stated that he never had been depressed his entire life. He remarked that he agreed to be tested just to make his wife happy. Two weeks later he committed suicide before his nutrient therapy for undermethylation had begun. Published studies indicate that 50% of depressed Americans never seek treatment. I believe a high percentage of these persons have the undermethylated biotype of depression.

Folate Deficiency Depression

About 20% of the 2,800 persons in my depression database exhibit folate deficiency as their primary nutrient imbalance. In general, they present a combination of symptoms and traits that distinguishes them from the other depression biotypes. Most report anxiety in addition to depression, and about 20% have a history of panic disorder or anxiety disorder. With very few exceptions, these persons report intolerance to SSRI antidepressants and antihistamines. A high percentage are noncompetitive persons who complain of chemical and food sensitivities but deny hay fever and other seasonal allergies. Despite their suffering, a surprising number are caring, generous persons with a history of volunteer work, and they probably are wonderful neighbors. The incidence of ADHD and academic underachievement is about three times higher than that observed for the undermethylated biotype. Table 6-3 presents symptoms and traits in high incidence for the low- folate biotype of depression.

Table 6-3.
Symptoms and Traits – Low-Folate Depression

-- Improvement after folate therapy	-- High anxiety and panic tendency
-- Adverse reaction to SSRIs	-- Improvement after benzodiazapines
-- Food and chemical sensitivities	-- Absence of seasonal allergies
-- Dry eyes and mouth	-- Low libido
-- High artistic abilities and interest	-- Hirsutism (males only)
-- Nervous legs, pacing	-- Sleep disorder
-- Noncompetitive in sports, games	-- Underachievement in school
-- Hyperactivity	-- High pain threshold
-- Upper body/head/neck pain	-- Adverse reaction to SAMe, methionine
-- Estrogen intolerance	-- Copper intolerance

Laboratory indications of low-folate depression include whole blood histamine below 40 ng/ml, an elevated SAMe/SAH ratio, low serum folate, and an absolute basophil count below 30. Diagnosis of this biotype is aided by the presence or absence of the factors shown in Table 6-3. The presence of 40% of the above symptoms and traits is consistent with the low-folate biotype of depression. Nutrient therapy for this biotype is focused on building up folate stores aimed at increasing acetylation of chromatin. Typical treatment formulations for low-folate depression include the following:

- Folic or folinic acid
- Vitamin B-12
- Niacinamide, choline, DMAE, and manganese that reduce dopamine synaptic activity
- Zinc, PLP, and vitamin B-6, which tend to increase GABA levels
- Augmenting nutrients, including vitamins C and E

It is also important to avoid supplements of tryptophan, 5-HTP, phenylalanine, tyrosine, copper, and inositol in treating these individuals. Originally, folic acid dosages exceeding two mg/day were routinely prescribed to combat low-folate depression. However, folinic acid more efficiently passes the blood-brain barrier, enabling lower folate dosages for this depression biotype.

Depression Case History 3 – Low Folate

Marilyn, age 36, is a slender, unmarried woman who arrived for her initial clinical evaluation wearing a face mask for protection against chemical allergies. Her medical history was obtained at an outdoor picnic table since she reacted to the chemicals in our new carpeting. Marilyn reported poor academics through elementary and high school despite an IQ of 132 and motivation to succeed. She was diagnosed with ADD in the fourth grade and took Ritalin until eighth grade. She said Ritalin helped with concentration but was discontinued after appetite suppression resulted in extreme weight loss.

Marilyn reported an onset of depression at age 20 while working as a waitress. She tried counseling for six months, but that didn't bear fruit. After taking Zoloft for two weeks, she reported severe worsening of depression and her first panic attack. Her doctor prescribed several other SSRI medications that also failed to provide benefits. However, she experienced lessening of anxiety after taking Klonapin and was still continuing this benzodiazepine medication. She reported other symptoms of low-folate depression including chemical sensitivities, problems concentrating, dry eyes, low libido, and chronic neck pain. She reported taking Benedryl on one occasion and feeling "wired" and agitated.

Marilyn's histamine tested at 16 ng/ml, and she was treated with high doses of folic acid, vitamin B-12, and niacinamide. Other prescribed nutrients included zinc, DMAE, manganese, chromium, and vitamins B-6, C and E, and she was urged to continue her Klonapin medication for several months. Marilyn complained of heightened anxiety after two weeks of therapy but reported significant improvement in depression and anxiety (but not chemical sensitivities) at a 4-month follow-up visit. Her treatment was fine-tuned, based on new lab work, and we suggested yearly checkups. The following year she reported improvement in all areas and no longer wore a face mask. Her Klonapin was discontinued by gradually reducing doses for several months. She has continued nutrient therapy for the past six years and reports being "95% better."

Depression Case History 4 – Low Folate

Karl, age 28, is a successful businessman in a Minnesota suburb, operating a family chemical business. He played football in high school but had been a below-average student. He stated he was happily married with two beautiful children. Karl said he had experienced brief episodes of depression as a teen, but severe anxiety, depression, and a sleep disorder developed at age 25. He saw a counselor at his church for more than a year, without significant improvement. He reported that Prozac provided some benefit but had to be discontinued due to nausea and headaches. Treatment with Paxil, Zoloft, and Celexa (SSRI medications) resulted in heightened anxiety and depression. Karl exhibited several symptoms of the low-folate biotype, including low libido, eye dryness that prevented wearing contact lenses, proficiency in water color painting, and thick hair on his chest and back. Karl's blood histamine level was 31 ng/ml, confirming his low folate status. His treatment centered on high doses of folic acid, vitamin B-12, and niacinamide. In addition, he received zinc, manganese, GABA, magnesium, DMAE, and vitamins B-6, C, and E. Karl has continued his nutrient therapy for several years and reports that he is quite well.

SSRI medications have benefited millions of depressed patients, but there are serious concerns about occasional persons who experience worsened depression or become violent after starting SSRIs. Persons with the low-folate biotype of depression are especially prone to these adverse side effects, presumably because they are intrinsically high-serotonin persons who react badly to medications that increase serotonin neurotransmission.

Depression Case History 5 – Low Folate

A middle-aged man from Colorado reported suicidal depression at his initial visit to our clinic. Concerned about his safety while waiting for lab results, we urged him to see a psychiatrist immediately after returning to Colorado. His wife later reported that her husband was given 20 mg/day of Prozac soon after returning home, but that the depression became sharply worse within a week. He returned to the psychiatrist who recognized lack of improvement and doubled the Prozac dosage. Six days later her husband committed suicide. Soon after hearing of his death, his lab results arrived showing histamine at 24 ng/ml, indicating the low-folate depression biotype associated with intolerance to SSRI medications.[108]

The school shootings at Columbine High School and Virginia Tech were carried out by students who had begun taking SSRI antidepressants.[109] The FDA has mandated that prescriptions for SSRIs contain a warning that "antidepressants increase the risk of suicidal thinking and behavior." It seems likely that persons with the low-folate biotype are especially vulnerable to this medication side effect. I recommend that psychiatrists perform simple blood tests prior to initiating SSRI therapy in order to identify low-folate individuals who are at high risk for adverse side effects.

Hypercupremic Depression

About 17% of depression patients exhibit hypercupremia or elevated copper (Cu) as their dominant chemical imbalance. The vast majority (96%) of persons with this biotype are women, with the first episode of depression typically occurring during a hormonal event such as puberty, childbirth, or menopause. In addition to depression, characteristic symptoms include severe anxiety, sleep disorder, hormone imbalances, hyperactivity in childhood, skin sensitivity to metals and rough fabrics, ringing in the ears (tinnitus), and intolerance to estrogen, shellfish, and chocolate.

In healthy persons, copper levels in blood and brain are homeostatically controlled through the actions of metallothionein and ceruloplasmin proteins.[32] This is essential for mental functioning since abnormal Cu levels can alter the amounts of dopamine and norepinephrine neurotransmitters in the brain as described in Chapter 3 (see Figure 3-1). Dopamine is often described as a "feel good" chemical that helps combat depression. Norepinephrine elevations have been associated with anxiety/panic disorders, sleep problems, paranoia, and, in severe cases, psychosis. Copper-overloaded depressives usually report that serotonin-enhancing antidepressants provide improvement in moods, but they worsen anxiety. Benzodiazapines such as Klonapin and Xanax can be effective in reducing anxiety but are reported to have little effect on depression for this biotype. High-copper females are usually intolerant of birth control pills or hormone replacement therapy since these treatments increase copper levels in the blood.

A straightforward way to treat persons with this depression biotype is to decopper them and bring blood and brain copper levels into the normal range. This can usually be achieved within 60 days using nutrient therapy. A primary natural mechanism for removal of excess copper involves binding to metallothionein (MT) proteins in the liver, followed by excretion via the bile duct. The genetic expression (production) of MT proteins is dependent on zinc, and this trace metal is usually depleted in high-copper persons. Accordingly, advanced nutrient therapy for reducing copper levels involves increasing MT protein levels using supplements of zinc together with manganese, glutathione, vitamins B-6, C, and E, and other nutrients known to increase MT activity. This therapy must be introduced gradually to avoid sudden release of excess copper into blood that could cause a temporary worsening of depression and anxiety. Patients currently taking psychiatric medications should continue them during the initial two to three months of nutrient therapy. However, more than 85% of high-copper patients report that psychiatric medication can eventually be eliminated without the return of depression.

An alternative decoppering therapy is the use of tetrathiomolybdate (TTM), which has been championed by Brewer and associates[110] for treatment of Wilson's disease and solid tumors. TTM can rapidly reduce copper levels without significant adverse side effects. Once copper levels have normalized, the TTM therapy can be replaced by zinc supplements, which stimulate production of MT proteins. This medication is still in the development stage. Trientine dihydrochloride and D-penicillamine are medications that effectively remove copper, but they usually involve serious adverse effects.

Elevated serum copper is exhibited by most women with a history of postpartum depression (PPD). Moreover, the classic symptoms of PPD are consistent with elevated norepinephrine and depleted dopamine that can result from copper overload. A large study[111] by Crayton and Walsh reported that depressed women with a history of PPD have significantly elevated serum copper when compared with depressed women without a history of PPD. Following decoppering nutrient therapy, most PPD patients exhibited normal concentrations of serum copper and reported major reductions in depression and anxiety.

PPD is a condition[73] occurring in the postnatal period that is characterized by depressed mood, lack of energy, disruptions of sleep, high anxiety, reduced interest in previously enjoyable activities, and, in severe cases, suicidal and homicidal ideation and behavior. Most women experience mild depressive symptoms soon after childbirth, and 10-20% will experience a full-blown depressive episode. Normal pregnancies involve greatly increased levels of estrogens and copper in blood. During the nine months of a normal pregnancy, serum copper typically doubles from about 110 mcg/

dl to about 220 mcg/dl. This additional copper enables rapid development of blood vessels (angiogenesis) needed for normal growth of the fetus. Normally, copper and estrogen levels begin to drop within 24 hours of delivery. It appears that PPD women have a genetic or acquired inability to eliminate excess copper. I have met hundreds of women with PPD who said that their depression began immediately after a pregnancy and persisted for years. Most of these women reported major improvements following nutrient therapy to normalize copper levels in blood. I have also met dozens of patients with postpartum psychosis that persisted for more than 20 years who reported major improvement after copper levels were normalized.

Depression Case History 6 – Hypercupremia

Kathleen, age 34, reported increasing depression following her first two pregnancies and suicidal depression after birth of her third child. Two years of counseling and psychiatric medications had failed to provide significant benefits. She said that her relationship with her husband had deteriorated and that minor stresses would reduce her to tears. Symptoms of copper overload included history of childhood hyperactivity, ringing in the ears, skin sensitivity to cheap metals, inability to tan, and severe worsening of depression after hormone therapy. Her serum copper level was 212 mcg/dl, compared to the normal range of 85-115 mcg/dl, and plasma zinc was out-of-range low at 65 mcg/dl. Initial treatment involved 25 mg/day of zinc, with the dose gradually increased to 75 mg/day. Kathleen complained of heightened anxiety during this period. Her complete program included ample amounts of B-6 and PLP together with supplements of manganese, DMAE, and vitamins B-3, C, and E. At her 6-month follow-up evaluation, Kathleen's metal levels had normalized and she reported that her depression was gone and that her marriage was solid again.

Depression Case History 7 – Hypercupremia

Carol, age 31, had been free of depression until she started birth control pills at age 16. Despite chronic depression, she excelled in college and had begun a successful career by age 24. She continued birth control after marriage and had never been pregnant. Carol stated that depression had become very severe with persistent thoughts of killing herself by crashing her car into a concrete viaduct. She was too embarrassed to have counseling but tried Effexor, Paxil, and Zoloft in the recent past without improvement. She exhibited symptoms of copper overload including intolerance to chocolate, allergy to shellfish, extreme skin sensitivity, and occasional rages.

Carol's lab results revealed elevated serum copper and depressed plasma zinc, and she was diagnosed with a metal metabolism disorder. Her therapy consisted of nutrients known to promote MT protein activity including zinc, manganese, selenium, DMAE, glutathione, 15 protein constituents of MT, and vitamins B-6, C, E, and PLP. Susan called several times during the first two weeks of nutrient therapy concerned that her depression appeared to be worsening. However, she noticed clear improvement during month two, and after six months she stated that she was depression free for the first time in eight years. We informed Carol that she was prone to postpartum depression and advised her to avoid prenatal vitamins containing copper if she became pregnant.

Pyroluric Depression

Approximately 15% of the 2,800 persons in our depression database exhibited elevated pyrroles as their dominant chemical imbalance. This is a stress disorder with onset of depression often triggered by severe emotional or physical trauma. These persons usually exhibit an odd combination of symptoms that makes diagnosis relatively straightforward. For example, most pyrolurics experience about 50% of the following symptoms and traits: severe mood swings, inability to cope with stress, rages, absence of dream recall, sunburn tendency and inability to tan, morning nausea, and sensitivity to bright lights and loud noises. As described in Chapter 5, many persons with severe pyrrole disorder have slender wrists, ankles, and neck, while having great amounts of fat at their midsection and upper thighs. Female pyrolurics may report disturbed menstrual periods or amenorrhea (absence of periods). Persons with this depression biotype are prone to delayed puberty and significant growth after age 16. Other symptoms include great inner tension, reading disorders, and academic underachievement regardless of intelligence. They tend to be fearful and pessimistic persons and isolate themselves from others. Many persons with this biotype are diagnosed with rapid-cycling bipolar disorder because of extreme mood swings that may occur many times daily. Most pyrolurics live in a world of fear and are obsessed with disasters such as the sinking of the Titanic, terrorist attacks, tornadoes, and earthquakes.

As described in Chapter 3, persons with pyrrole disorder suffer from a double deficiency of zinc and vitamin B-6 that may be genetic in nature. This results in a tendency for low brain levels of serotonin, dopamine, and GABA, which is a recipe for depression and anxiety. Nutrient therapy for pyrrole disorder simply involves normalization of zinc and B-6 levels. Deficiencies of zinc and B-6 may be severe and genetic in nature, and high doses (many times the RDA) are often required to bring blood zinc and B-6 to normal levels. Pyrrole disorders indicate elevated oxidative stress: ample dosages of selenium, glutathione, vitamin C, vitamin E, and other antioxidants assist in treatment. Depressed persons with pyrrole disorder respond more quickly to nutrient therapy than the other depression biotypes. Clear improvement is usually noticed within a few days, with the therapy achieving full effect within four to six weeks.

Because of morning nausea, many persons with pyrrole disorder cannot tolerate nutrients until lunchtime. They tend to perform badly in morning and are at their best late at night. Some observers believe the legend of Dracula originated from violent pyrolurics who were very sensitive to light and thrived at night. My database studies indicate a very high incidence of pyrrole disorder is found in persons diagnosed with antisocial personality disorder, previously known as sociopaths (see Chapter 8). Fortunately most pyrolurics do not have criminal tendencies. The following are case histories that illustrate the diagnosis and treatment of the pyrrole disorder biotype of depression.

Depression Case History 8 – Pyrrole Disorder

Curt, age 24, had been a star football player in high school, but he was a below-average student. He disliked academics and took a job with the railroad after graduation. He was famous for his temper and had several arrests for assault. Curt complained of chronic depression and suicidal ideation since the age of 16. He was muscular with Hollywood good looks and had a very engaging personality. He was interested in girls but seldom dated because of embarrassing erectile dysfunction. He had been terminated from two jobs for physically assaulting his supervisor. Curt was late for his initial appointment due to a physical altercation with a state trooper who stopped him for speeding. He reported several symptoms consistent with pyrrole disorder, including internal tension, poor short-term memory, absence of dream recall, enjoyment of spicy foods, pale complexion, avoidance of breakfast, and sensitivity to sunlight.

Curt's lab chemistries were unremarkable except for urine pyrroles that were 10 times above the normal level. His nutrient therapy involved powerful doses of vitamin B-6 and zinc along with augmenting nutrients aimed at lessening oxidative stress (selenium, manganese, vitamins C, and E). After two weeks of nutrient therapy, Curt called to report that he felt "weird" and was concerned that the vitamins were changing his personality. He was experiencing internal calm for the first time in his life and was alarmed at the striking change. At a 3-month check-up visit, Curt reported his depression had disappeared along with his violent temper but that the erectile dysfunction problem remained. For the past several years he has continued the nutrient therapy and reports that Viagra has normalized his social life. He has held a steady job and had no episodes of depression or police contacts during this period.

Depression Case History 9 – Pyrrole Disorder

Marianne, age 32, was unmarried and living with her parents in a Chicago suburb. She reported a troubled childhood that included special education and treatment for depression and intermittent explosive disorder. She was mainstreamed in high school but had few friends and was at the bottom of most classes academically. She received counseling from social workers and a psychologist for several years that was helpful, but she often relapsed during stressful periods. After high school, she had several minimum wage jobs but was chronically unemployed. Her depression and emotional outbursts continued despite treatment by three psychiatrists who prescribed more than a dozen psychiatric medications in an attempt to help her.

Eventually Marianne's parents sought nutrient therapy that they referred to as a last resort. She exhibited several symptoms of pyrrole disorder, including abnormal menstrual cycles, inability to handle stress, wild mood swings, white spots on fingernails, and morning nausea. In addition, she wore dark sunglasses throughout daytime hours and stated that she had never experienced a dream. Her urine sample turned a reddish-purple mauve color during storage in the lab refrigerator, and her pyrrole level tested at 82 mcg/dl. Marianne was diagnosed with severe pyrrole disorder and was treated with strong doses of vitamin B-6, PLP, and zinc in conjunction with augmenting nutrients aimed at reducing oxidative stress. She experienced early compliance problems, so her nutrients were compounded to reduce the number of capsules.

Marianne's parents reported that she underwent a transformation over the next four months. They were especially pleased that she appeared much happier, and her emotional outbursts had ceased. Two years later, we learned that Marianne had a steady job and was living independently in an apartment. She reported that she had been quite well and was faithfully continuing the nutrient therapy. Marianne said that she still felt uncomfortable in social situations, and we suggested that counseling might help.

Toxic Overload Depression

Approximately 5% of the 2,800 persons in our depression database exhibited toxic-metal poisoning as their primary chemical imbalance. Most of these cases involved overloads of lead, mercury, cadmium, or arsenic. This form of depression is estimated to affect one in every 500 persons, corresponding to more than 600,000 cases in the USA. Common features of this depression biotype are the following:

- Depression that arises suddenly during a period of relative calm and wellness
- Abdominal pain and cramping
- Increased irritability
- Headaches and muscle weakness
- Low energy
- Failure to respond to counseling or psychiatric medications

Toxic metal overload can be difficult to diagnose due to low concentrations of toxic metals in blood. An example of metal toxicity that does not usually show up in a blood test applies to the case of mercury: after a very short number of days, elevated mercury will not be found in the blood, having moved to other body tissues such as fatty tissue. Since depression due to metal toxicity is relatively uncommon, a logical first step is to rule out the presence of undermethylation, folate deficiency, copper overload, pyrrole disorder, casein/gluten allergy, or a thyroid imbalance. A careful chemical analysis of toxic metals in scalp hair can serve as a screen, recognizing the possibility of a false positive resulting from external contamination. Many doctors test for toxic metal overload by introducing a chelating chemical that drives toxins from the body and then measuring the increased amount of toxins being excreted in the stool and urine. Unfortunately, reliable reference ranges have not yet been established for these challenge tests. Another barrier to diagnosis is differing symptoms for the various toxic metals. However, when depression due to toxic metals is accurately diagnosed, nutrient therapy can usually provide significant benefits.

Young children are especially sensitive to toxic metals since their blood-brain barriers are still immature, and the toxins can interfere with the development of brain cells and receptors. For example, lead poisoning can reduce IQ in young children but has little effect on the mental capability of an adult. Depression, irritability, abdominal discomfort, kidney damage, and liver damage are the primary results of serious metal poisoning for adults. Toxic metals in the brain can cause great mischief including the following:

+ weakening of the blood-brain barrier
+ altered neurotransmitter levels
+ destruction or demyelination of the myelin sheath
+ increased oxidative stress
+ destruction of glutathione and other protective proteins

It is, therefore, not surprising that a toxic metal overload can cause clinical depression.

Nutrient therapy for lead poisoning involves supplements of calcium, promotion of metallothionein synthesis, and generous supplementation of antioxidants. Lead is a bone seeker with about 95% of old lead stored within the skeletal structure.[112] In the absence of therapies to remove lead, the half-life of lead in humans is estimated at 22 years. Nutrient therapy and chelation techniques can effectively remove lead from blood and soft tissues but cannot rapidly remove lead from bone. Persons with high levels of lead in their bones are continuously exposed to this toxin as it slowly departs the skeletal system. Accordingly, these persons may need to continue therapy to remove lead for the rest of their lives. In most cases, this can be accomplished by inexpensive supplements of calcium and zinc. However, many calcium supplements have significant impurity levels of lead, and care should be taken to obtain high-purity products.

Depression Case History 10 – Toxic Overload

John, age 54, developed severe depression during a 12-month leave of absence from his job in downtown Chicago. He reported that counseling and several antidepressants had absolutely no effect on his condition. He also complained of uncharacteristic anger, nausea, and abdominal cramping. John's lab chemistries were unremarkable except for a blood lead level 80 times above the normal level. I asked John to return to the clinic for an impromptu conference. He returned that afternoon covered from head to toe with flecks of paint. John said he had purchased a beautiful old house and had spent the past six months scraping paint from the interior walls. At the time of my call, he was on a scaffold scraping paint off the outside of the house. We concluded that he had poisoned himself with repeated exposure to lead-based paint. A second blood test confirmed the diagnosis of lead poisoning. Since his depression was severe, he was hospitalized for several days and received EDTA chelation. Within a week, John reported that his depression was completely gone and that he decided to sell his house. We prescribed supplements of calcium, zinc, selenium, and vitamins C and E to protect against lead that would be slowly leaching from his bones.

Mercury is a lethal poison that is especially devastating to children from conception to age four years, the period when most brain development occurs. The half-life of mercury in the periphery of the body (everything except the brain) is about 42 days.[112] The half-life of mercury in the brain has been measured at 70 days. However, mercury half-lives may be much higher for persons with a genetic metal metabolism disorder or severe oxidative stress. Mercury has a remarkable affinity for glutathione and MT proteins, and nutrient therapy that increases amounts of these proteins can effectively remove mercury from the body. Chelation and other therapies have been under active development for removal of mercury from autistic children. It is impossible to totally eliminate mercury exposure since each day we receive about 1 microgram (mcg) of mercury from breathing and another 10-20 mcg from a typical diet. A meal involving tuna or other large fish may bring an additional 20-40 mcg. Healthy persons have protective proteins that bind to mercury and render it harmless. However, some individuals have a genetic weakness in this protective system and may be extremely vulnerable to even modest mercury exposures.

Cadmium[112] is especially dangerous since it tends to accumulate at kidney tubules and cause permanent damage. Sources of cadmium include shellfish, shallow wells, fertilizers, metal welding, brazing, fireworks, artist's paints, mining operations, and various industrial plants. Cadmium is present in cigarettes, and smoking one to two packs daily can double blood and tissue levels of the metal. Cadmium removal must be accomplished with caution to avoid kidney damage, and treatments that enhance MT proteins are safer than chelation therapies that divert the departing cadmium through the kidneys.

Arsenic overloads are relatively rare and difficult to diagnose. The symptoms include upper respiratory problems, anorexia, muscle weakness, and irritation of mucous membranes. A definitive test for arsenic poisoning is the presence of elevated levels in both urine and scalp hair. Unfortunately, reference normals for these assays are poorly defined, and interpretation of the results involves a degree of speculation. The biological half-lives of arsenic compounds are brief, ranging from 10 to 30 hours. The principal sources of arsenic are seafoods, contaminated drinking water, and pesticides. It has also been found on treated wood and playground equipment and in poultry feed. Nutrient therapy involving calcium and enhancement of glutathione protein levels can hasten the exit of arsenic. These therapies are seldom useful for single environmental exposures since arsenic leaves the body quickly and may be at safe levels before treatment can begin. However, depressed persons living (or working) in high arsenic environments may benefit from nutrient supplements that protect against arsenic toxicity.

Mainstream Medicine and Depression Biotypes

Despite brilliant advances in brain science, mainstream medicine continues to regard clinical depression as a single entity rather than a collection of different disorders. Dysthymia, postpartum depression, seasonal affective disorder, and other types of depression are believed to be variations within a central theme: low serotonin neurotransmission kinetics. Consequently, most persons diagnosed with depression are initially treated with SSRI medications aimed at increasing serotonin activity. The SSRI antidepressants can benefit persons with the undermethylation or pyrrole biotypes of depression but can harm folate-deficient depressives and be ineffective for the other biotypes. Treatment outcomes could be greatly improved if physicians would order inexpensive blood tests to identify the patients who are good candidates for SSRI antidepressants. Additional benefits could be achieved if nutrient imbalances associated with the different depression biotypes were diagnosed and treated. It's likely that nutrient therapy would improve SSRI treatment outcomes, including reduction or elimination of adverse side effects. In many cases, nutrient therapy alone could prove to be effective.

CHAPTER 7

AUTISM

Introduction

In 1939, Winston Churchill referred to Russia as "a riddle wrapped in a mystery inside an enigma." Today these words could be used to describe autism. First reported by psychiatrist Leo Kanner[113-114] in 1943, autism spectrum disorders have reached epidemic proportions, increasing from 3 in 10,000 births to about 1 in 100 in the USA.[115] A typical schoolteacher in the period 1940 to 1980 encountered one or two cases in an entire career. Today most teachers learn of new autism cases in their districts each month. For several decades, the increasing numbers were attributed to better efficiency of diagnosis. However, this cannot explain the continuing sharp increases since 1990 when the syndrome of autism became well known throughout the medical field.

Genetics, Epigenetics, and Environment

There is an undeniable heritable component to autism, with about 60-90% concordance in identical twins in contrast to less than 10% for fraternal twins.[116] Since concordance is less than 100%, a very significant environmental component exists. I once studied an autistic adult with wild behavior and severe cognitive delays, and then I met his identical twin who was a personable, highly successful professional. They had identical physical appearance and blood/urine chemistry, but the difference in their level of functioning was staggering. The mother said both sons developed normally the first 18 months, after which one twin developed severe autism symptoms while the other continued to thrive. She had no explanation for the difference in her sons. Another case involved identical twin boys (age 3) who presented with very similar autism symptoms and biochemistry. After a few years of biochemical treatment, one twin achieved a full recovery and has been excelling in a mainstream classroom. His brother had a partial improvement but is still on the autism spectrum. Since their treatments and diets were identical for years, it seems likely one twin experienced more severe environmental insults, such as exposure to pesticides or toxic metals.

Many people ask, "How can there be an epidemic of a genetic disorder?" And, in fact, there cannot be a purely genetic epidemic. Heritable DNA mutations usually require centuries to develop. Spontaneous DNA abnormalities in human beings occur about once in every 500,000 cell divisions, and few are transferred to the next generation. As described in Chapter 4, fetal development during the first month of pregnancy is sensitive to environmental insults that can disrupt epigenetic processes that govern which genes are expressed and which are silenced. These epigenetic abnormalities usually persist throughout life, and, in certain cases, may be passed on to future generations. In any case, it is clear that the increased rates of autism are due to changes in the environment over the past 70 years. More than two-dozen theories have been suggested, including increased vaccinations, toxic metal exposures (also possible via vaccines), changes in the water supply, a compromised in utero environment, industrial food processing, and changes in family dynamics. There is little agreement among autism researchers and clinicians regarding the environmental triggers, but one thing has become very clear: the usual recipe for autism is a combination of an inherited predisposition and severe environmental insults prior to age three.

Autism Onset

Approximately four out of every five children diagnosed with autism are male. Until 1960, most cases involved clear symptoms at birth. During the ensuing decades, *regressive autism* rates gradually increased and now represent about 80% of cases.[117] The reason(s) for the increased prevalence of regressive autism is still being debated. In typical regression cases, children develop normally until age 16-24 months, when a fairly sudden decline in functioning occurs.

I have met hundreds of parents who reported their child had developed normally until they approached age two. In a typical case, the child was in good health, happy, and beginning to speak when an unexpected regression occurred over a few days or weeks. Most families reported loss of speech; a divergent gaze; odd, repetitive movements; disinterest in parents and siblings; gastrointestinal symptoms; and emotional meltdowns. A visit to the pediatrician usually was followed by evaluation at a child development center. Many families tearfully described their horror at receiving a diagnosis of autism and being told the condition was incurable and would result in a lifetime of severe handicap. This scenario is still common today, and many families are advised to institutionalize their child, despite the fact that many children are recovering—losing their autism classification and becoming indistinguishable from their same-age peers—with appropriate, individualized interventions.

The Dark Ages of Autism—1945 to 1975

The psychiatry profession has provided great benefits to society over the past century. However, mainstream psychiatry's theories regarding autism were dead wrong for about 30 years, resulting in lack of scientific progress and failed therapeutic approaches. Leo Kanner's first publication in 1943 described autism as a severe developmental disorder caused by poor parenting.[113] He summarized 11 case histories and reported that all of the parents were uncaring and lacking in empathy. Kanner concluded that these children had been emotionally deprived during the early years, resulting in enduring deficits in socialization and communication. A popular early treatment involved isolating the children from their "incompetent" parents, and showering them with affection and encouragement in an institutional setting. This well-intentioned—but ineffective—approach persisted for decades. In 1967, famed autism expert Bruno Bettelheim of the University of Chicago published a book[118] titled *The Empty Fortress: Infantile Autism and the Birth of the Self* that influenced autism therapists for several decades. Bettelheim claimed that autism was the result of a "refrigerator mother" who wished the child had never been born and a weak or absent father.

My first experience with autism involved a research colleague whose only child was diagnosed with autism in the 1960s. When we became close friends, he confided that he and his wife were being treated for clinical depression that began upon learning of their son's autism, and the depression dramatically worsened after experts explained they were failures as parents and had caused their son's disorder. During this time period, countless thousands of parents suffered great anguish when the finger of blame was pointed directly at them. The world now knows that the concept of a refrigerator mother and distant father was completely wrong and did great harm. In fact, the exact opposite is true. Most parents of children diagnosed with autism are remarkably loving and extremely dedicated to helping their child.

A misguided belief that still persists is that autism is incurable and affected children face a dismal future. Recent advances in biomedical and behavioral therapies have resulted in thousands of reports of recovery throughout the world. Most of these reports involved intervention prior to age four, but significant progress can be made at any age. I once received a phone call from a mother from Connecticut who said her 17-year-old daughter began speaking after two months of biochemical therapy! (Biochemical therapy, which uses chemicals natural to the body, is a subset of biomedical therapy.) Medical science is sometimes slow to adopt new effective therapies, and lack of compelling scientific evidence—the funding and publication of which is prey to political roadblocks—is often part of the problem. I look forward to the time when the medical and scientific communities acknowledge that *autism is treatable*, and parents of affected children are urged to seek aggressive (yet safe) treatment immediately after diagnosis.

Symptoms and Traits

There is an old saying that "Once you've met one autistic child, you've met one autistic child." There is great variation in symptoms and traits from child to child. Some are hyperactive, and others are lethargic. Many are completely nonverbal, whereas others have significant speech. About 30% have abnormal EEG brain waves and a tendency for seizures. Some have explosive behavior, and others are quite calm. Despite these individual differences, there are classic symptoms and traits usually present in four key areas.[73]

+ *Socialization:* This includes very poor social skills, including lack of interest in others, resistance to cuddling and holding, and an apparent preference to retreat into their own world.

+ *Language:* This includes either absence of speech or a major speech delay, inability to start a conversation or keep one going, a tendency to repeat the sounds of others (echolalia), an unusual tone or rhythm of speech, and a very limited expressive vocabulary.

+ *Behavior:* This category includes repetitive movements, such as rocking, spinning or hand flapping; behavioral routines or rituals; little or no eye contact; an obsessive interest in certain objects, such as spinning toys, or using the parts of toys in an atypical way (e.g., perseverating on spinning the car wheels); an inability to make transitions; sensitivity to touch, light, and sounds; and impulsive actions, such as running into the street.

+ *Cognition:* This involves slowness in acquiring new knowledge or skills and weakness in applying knowledge to everyday life.

In addition, a high percentage of children diagnosed with autism have significant physical problems, including poor immune function, severe constipation, food allergies, intestinal yeast overgrowth, and heightened sensitivity to toxic metals. These fall under broader physiological issues that include oxidative stress, immune dysregulation, and detoxification impairment.

Differential Diagnosis

Autism spectrum disorders consist of three major types: (1) classical or Kanner's autism, (2) pervasive developmental disorder—not otherwise specified (PDD-NOS), and (3) Asperger's disorder (aka Asperger's syndrome).[73] There are great differences in severity among the three groups. Asperger's syndrome is often referred to as high-functioning autism and typically involves normal or above-normal intelligence and competent speech. However, Asperger's individuals exhibit very poor socialization, divergent gaze, atypical behaviors, and obsessive or ritualistic interests. Many are savants with extraordinary abilities in mathematics, memory, or music. Dustin Hoffman's character in the movie *Rain Man* provides an excellent example of Asperger's syndrome.

Classical or Kanner's autism is the most severe disorder in the autism spectrum, and its sufferers usually exhibit most of the above symptoms and traits by age three. Without effective treatment, these individuals are likely to experience a lifetime of frustration and unhappiness as well as severe deficits in cognition, socialization, and speech. Fortunately, advanced biochemical therapies usually result in exciting partial progress, with many reports of complete recovery. There is a great need for controlled scientific studies to accurately measure effectiveness of these new therapies. Such studies are hampered by the very high placebo rate (about 40%) in autism, perhaps arising from an inability to control the environment of children who are highly sensitive to a multitude of factors (known and unknown). In many cases, placebo effects do not involve imaginary improvements but actual improvements that have nothing to do with the treatment. In addition, it is difficult to recruit families if their child might be in a control group that uses the placebo.

Children diagnosed with PDD-NOS have symptoms that are intermediate in severity between classical autism and Asperger's syndrome. The distinction between classical autism and PDD-NOS is not always clear, and many children receive both diagnoses after evaluation by separate professionals. A large chemistry database study in 2001 reported very disordered blood and urine chemistries for all members of the autism spectrum, with no detectable difference between classical autism, PDD-NOS, and Asperger's.[119] This finding suggests that all members of the autism spectrum may have the same inherited predisposition but differ in the type, severity, or timing of environmental insults. For example, children who achieve a higher degree of brain development prior to the insults would be expected to be capable of higher functioning.

The Autistic Regression Event

Although experts are able to detect subtle autism tendencies by studying early video tapes, the extreme deterioration that often occurs within a few days needs explanation. I have met hundreds of parents who reported very rapid regressions, including cases in which vaccinations, illnesses, or known toxic exposures were not involved. The global nature of the regressions can be striking, including loss of speech, odd repetitive movements, divergent gaze, sudden intolerance to certain foods, and extreme personality change. It seems clear that a major *event* has occurred within the brain—and perhaps throughout the entire body.

Wilson's disease[73] and schizophrenia are other medical conditions that involve a rapid deterioration in cognitive functioning after a period of relative normalcy. An important difference is that autism develops during a critical early phase of brain development. The median age of onset of Wilson's disease is 17 years. In this disorder, the ability to remove copper from the liver and other organs is impaired, resulting in extreme deterioration in physical and mental functioning. Wilson's disease, schizophrenia, and autism are similar in that all involve oxidative overload, with extreme depletions of protective proteins MT and GSH. In Wilson's, gradual worsening of oxidative stress can progress until the MT and GSH antioxidant functions are overwhelmed, resulting in (a) sudden impairment of bile transport of copper from the liver and (b) dramatic worsening of symptoms.

The onset of schizophrenia usually occurs after age 16 during a period of severe emotional or physical stress that may increase oxidative overload and trigger the mental breakdown event. These similarities suggest that a study of the regressions in Wilson's disease and schizophrenia could provide valuable clues to the origin of autism spectrum disorders.

The extreme suddenness of autistic regressions raises many intriguing questions, but the permanence of the autistic condition is even more mysterious. In the absence of early biochemical therapy, autism most often leads to a lifetime of disability. After age six, therapies that effectively overcome oxidative stress, toxic overloads, food sensitivities, yeast overload, metal metabolism imbalance, and weak immune function can provide significant improvements, but the essential autistic condition of cognitive and/or social and/or speech impairment usually remains at some level. I have witnessed hundreds of cases of autism recovery, but nearly all involved aggressive intervention prior to age four. This strongly suggests that (a) the central problem in autism is early brain development that has gone awry, and (b) a full recovery is extremely unlikely unless treatment begins before completion of this critical stage of brain maturation. Autism researchers and clinicians disagree on many points, but they unanimously agree that early intervention is essential. Medical institutions, government agencies, and insurance companies should rally to make this available to children immediately after diagnosis. Although early intervention is the most optimal route, there have been recoveries and major improvements—such as verbalization beginning in adulthood—that have occurred even when biomedical therapies were begun well after early childhood. Every individual with autism deserves our best dedicated efforts to improve their quality of life.

Findings Concerning Brain Structure

Many of the mysteries shrouding this illness have begun to be solved by autism researchers. Some of the more important findings involve differences in brain structure and organization. German researchers[120] have found anatomical abnormalities of the amygdala-fusiform system, indicating poor connectivity between these brain areas. Researchers at Harvard[121-122] and elsewhere have reported that primitive areas of autistic brains are immature, having failed to complete development of brain cells and synaptic connections. This knowledge suggests that therapies aimed at completion of brain development may be a high priority. Casanova[123-124] has reported abnormalities in the cortex of autistic brains, especially narrowing of minicolumn arrays of cells. McGinnis and colleagues[125] have reported threadlike accumulations of damaged fats in autistic brains, indicating oxidative damage. Courchesne[126] found that many children with autism experience a rapid acceleration in brain size during the first year of life. Approximately 25% of autistics develop unusually large heads during early development. All of these findings suggest that early intervention is of critical importance since brain abnormalities that develop in the initial years may persist throughout life. The plasticity of brain cells and synapses is greatest in infancy and early childhood, and exciting progress is possible during this window of time.

We all start life with billions of short, dense, brain cells that are immature. Brain development involves four basic phases:

1. Pruning of some brain cells to make space for growth of other cells
2. Growth of neurons, axons, dendrites, and other cell components
3. Growth inhibition once a brain cell is fully mature
4. Development of synaptic connections

Researchers have reported an excessive number of short, undeveloped brain cells in the cerebellum, pineal gland, hippocampus, and amygdala of individuals with autism. This brain immaturity is primarily in areas with little or no protection from the blood-brain barrier, suggesting that chemical insults or excessive oxidative stress may have stunted brain development. In addition, these children exhibit a poverty of dendrites and synaptic connections. The number of brain cells in a typical human brain is roughly equal to the number of trees in the United States; the number of dendrites has been likened to the number of leaves on those trees. In autism there are a reduced number of developed brain cells and fewer branches on the cells. The net result is a lessened ability to develop synaptic connections needed for learning, speech, and socialization.

The brain area with the most pronounced immaturity in autism is the cerebellum, which is responsible for smooth, controlled movements. A majority of individuals with autism exhibit odd, repetitive movements, possibly due to an impaired cerebellum. Another affected brain area is the amygdala that enables a person to develop social skills. Deficits in socialization are a hallmark of autism, and an immature amygdala may be part of the problem. The hippocampus partners with Wernieke's area and Broca's area in the development of speech. Mutism and speech delay are common in autism, and a poorly functioning hippocampus may be responsible.

Fortunately, the ability to develop immature brain cells and new synapses continues throughout life. This capability enables many paralyzed stroke victims to recover and also offers hope for children with autism. The speed with which new brain cells and synapses are developed is extremely rapid until about age four when a gradual slowing occurs. This explains why a four-year-old visiting Paris may speak fluent French within six weeks, while a teenager may require a year or more, and a senior citizen might never achieve this capability. Clinicians working with autistic children are aware of the critical need for early intervention. In my experience, greater progress can be achieved in one month with a two-year-old, than in six months with an eight-year-old. Doctors and parents need to be aware that immediate action is essential once the diagnosis of autism has been made.

Brains of individuals with autism also appear to be afflicted with significant inflammation[127] that may inhibit brain development and cause a myriad of symptoms, including irritability, speech delay, sleep disorders, cognitive delay, and increased head size. The sudden regression experienced by many children may be caused by events that result in brain inflammation.

High-Frequency Health Problems in Autism

In addition to the brain being structurally impacted, most children diagnosed with ASD experience physical problems[128] that can bring considerable misery to the child and make parenting very difficult. Many are afflicted with severe GI tract problems, including malabsorption, food sensitivities, esophagitis, reflux, incomplete digestion of proteins, yeast overgrowth, constipation, parasite overloads, and an incompetent intestinal barrier. Other common problems include poor immune function, seizures, sleep disturbances, chemical sensitivities, poor appetite, sensitivity to touch and sound, and enuresis (involuntary urination). There are numerous reports of high anxiety, apparent pain, frustration, and emotional meltdowns. Caregivers and educators would do well to first look to underlying physiological conditions that cause pain and other symptoms before attributing challenging behaviors to purely behavioral roots.

Many parents report their child's autism started immediately after a vaccination, and this is a hotly debated issue today. Most mainstream medical experts deny this relationship, but a genetic or acquired hypersensitivity to certain vaccines or an impaired ability to detoxify vaccine components remains a definite possibility. Another controversial and widespread belief is that autism is caused by exposure to mercury and other toxic metals. A 1999 FDA recommendation called for reducing or eliminating the mercury-containing preservative (Thimerosal) in childhood vaccinations. This has resulted in a major reduction of mercury exposures in the USA, although the elimination of mercury exposures to children is far from complete. Notwithstanding, autism rates have continued to escalate since the FDA's action,[115] suggesting that mercury is not the only suspect in autism causation. However, mercury is a highly poisonous substance, and the recommendation to remove Thimerosol from vaccines was a sensible public health measure.

The multiplicity of autism symptoms has hampered the ability to measure treatment effectiveness in clinical experiments. ASD children are highly sensitive to their environment, and there is continual waxing and waning of some symptoms due to changing conditions that may be imperceptible to the family. As a result, virtually every treatment approach will result in numerous reports of improvement. The result is that several ineffective therapies have gained popularity, and potentially effective therapies may have escaped notice. In autism research studies, the percent of improvement in control groups is usually greater than 40%, which presents a significant barrier to accurate evaluation of new therapies. Another research problem is that most ASD children have a history of aggressive therapy interventions that can alter the underlying condition. This has led some researchers to restrict their experiments to treatment naïve ASD children who have never been treated. Finally, what helps one child may not help another at a given time because of the order in which the interventions were done. For example, educational strategies work better after biochemical or other dietary therapies have already been initiated.

Food sensitivities

For several years, we tested for gluten and casein intolerance by measuring casomorphin and gluteomorphin levels in blood. These abnormal proteins result from incomplete breakdown of certain dairy and grain proteins in the digestive tract. There is considerable evidence that these deviant proteins can readily pass intestinal and brain barriers and cause a myriad of behavioral and cognitive problems. Children diagnosed with these food sensitivities were routinely placed on strict gluten-free/casein-free (GF/CF) diets. A study of 500 autism cases showed that 85% of families adopting the special diet reported major benefits. Hundreds of parents told me of very rapid and striking improvements in their children. A study of the 15% nonresponders revealed that about half had a family history of Crohn's disease or other inflammatory bowel disorder. This experience has convinced me that all autism spectrum children deserve a trial of the GF/CF diet, with or without the benefit of special laboratory testing.

Abnormal biochemistry

Children with autism exhibit distinctive chemical imbalances not present in the general population. By 1999, I had collected a database of 50,000 chemical assays of blood and urine for autistic children and was invited by the late Dr. Bernard Rimland of the Autism Research Institute to present the findings at a think tank in Cherry Hill, New Jersey. The assembled audience of autism researchers and clinicians was familiar with my findings:

- Zinc deficiency
- Copper overload
- B-6 deficiency
- Elevated toxic metals

However, the group expressed great surprise at data indicating that more than 90% of autistics were undermethylated. Subsequent research by S. Jill James,[69] Richard Deth,[70] and others has shown that undermethylation is a distinctive feature of autism. By 2009, a wealth of biochemical information had been collected by autism researchers throughout the world. Table 7-1 lists typical biochemical features of autism spectrum disorders.

Table 7-2 lists popular biomedical therapies aimed at normalizing body/brain chemistry in ASD patients. These treatment approaches have resulted in hundreds of reports of significant improvement, and each has developed a cadre of enthusiastic supporters. However, in every case, the treatment must be regarded as unproven until careful double-blind, placebo-controlled studies can prove efficacy. At present, none of these approaches has been adopted by mainstream medicine.

Table 7-1.
Biochemical Features of Autism (partial list)

- Low levels of glutathione
- Undermethylation
- Elevated mercury, lead, and other toxins
- Copper overload and insufficient ceruloplasmin
- Zinc deficiency
- Vitamin A deficiency
- Elevated urine pyrroles
- Depressed metallothionein protein levels
- Elevated carboxyethylpyrroles
- Low levels of magnesium
- Deficiency of selenium and cysteine

Oxidative stress

While evaluating extensive blood and urine chemistries for thousands of ASD patients, I learned that more than 99% exhibit evidence of excessive oxidative stress.[119] Chemical biomarkers for this condition include pervasive zinc deficiency; elevated pyrroles; low Cu/Zn SOD;[129] copper overload; low ceruloplasmin; undermethylation; low levels of glutathione, selenium, and MT proteins; and elevated levels of mercury, lead, and other toxic metals. Recent research studies have heightened interest in this area, and many experts now believe that oxidative stress is central to the etiology of autism.

Examination of the popular biochemical therapies shown in Table 7-2 reveals that nearly all provide an antioxidant effect. For example, the most commonly prescribed drug for autism patients is Risperdal, which has antioxidant properties. Therapies to overcome hypomethylation result in more robust levels of the natural antioxidants glutathione, MT proteins, and cysteine. The GF/CF diet results in reduced inflammation, which lowers antioxidant requirements.

Many respected researchers and clinicians believe that mercury poisoning is the central problem in autism and use chelating chemicals that strip this toxin out of the body. Chelation is a standard medical procedure used by mainstream medicine for cases of severe lead or mercury poisoning. We encountered several cases of toxic metal poisoning in depressed patients, and we were very impressed by the rapid and permanent recoveries following four or five days of in-hospital chelation therapy. However, I've learned that chelation of children with autism usually presents a

---

Table 7-2.
Popular Biomedical Therapies for Autism (partial list)[126]

- Methyl-B$_{12}$ and other methylation therapies
- Supplementation with vitamins/minerals found in deficiency
- Transdermal glutathione
- Casein-free, gluten-free diets
- Chelation (removal of toxic metals)
- Metallothionein-Promotion therapy
- N-Acetylcysteine and alpha lipoic acid
- Therapies to combat yeast overgrowth
- Antibacterials and antifungals
- Decoppering protocols
- Amino acid supplements
- Digestive enzymes
- Hormonal treatments
- Secretin
- Hyperbaric therapy

---

very different picture. In the late 1990s, we surveyed hundreds of families with an ASD child who had utilized chelation. In most cases, they reported very exciting improvements in their child during early stages of the therapy. Most parents said the improvements began to fade away after two to three weeks, with their child returning to the pretreatment condition. Many doctors concluded they needed to remove more mercury, and the 5-10 day chelation procedure was repeated. I met several families who had repeated this process more than 20 times over more than a year with the same result: definite improvement that faded away after about 17 days. It was clear to me that most of the excess mercury should have been removed after the first few chelations, and I concluded that the primary benefit was the powerful antioxidant effect of the chelating agent(s) rather than mercury removal. My chemical studies of thousands of children with autism revealed most to have high-normal levels of mercury but not mercury poisoning. High-normal toxic metal levels can result from weak antioxidant capability, without unusual mercury exposures. We did encounter a few autistic children with severe mercury poisoning, and a few weeks of oral DMSA chelation were administered to correct this problem.

Weakness in antioxidant protection makes individuals with autism especially sensitive to mercury, and the 1999 recommendation to remove mercury preservatives in childhood vaccinations was a sensible public health action. It must be noted that mercury can have a devastating effect on a developing brain. All families need to be vigilant in protecting their children from sources of toxic metals, including untested well water, contaminated toys, and lead-based paints. Even more important may be the need to avoid exposure to toxins during pregnancy. The bottom line is that elimination of excess oxidative stress is a requirement of an effective autism therapy program.

Seizures

Roughly one-third of children diagnosed with an autism spectrum disorder have a history of either seizures or abnormal electroencephalograms (EEGs). A careful study of 503 ASD children that excluded subjects with a history of seizure tendencies found about 99% to have copper and zinc imbalances. Several studies of ASD populations that include subjects with seizure tendencies reveal that a substantial number of ASD children do not exhibit these imbalances. This suggests that the combination of ASD and seizures may represent a phenotype that is distinctly different from other ASD children.

What Can a Family Do?

When a child is diagnosed with ASD, most families begin an intensive study of the disorder and quickly learn that early intervention is essential. The problem is that there are a multitude of treatments, and it is impossible to do all of them. The first decision is whether to limit therapy to the recommendations of mainstream medicine. After involvement with thousands of ASD patients, I've learned that most families are initially told that autism is incurable, and the most common recommendations are applied behavior analysis (ABA), Risperdal, and/or institutionalization. Most families who utilized ABA reported that this system helped their child, although the benefits were painstakingly slow, expensive, and quite limited. Risperdal is an atypical antipsychotic medication developed for schizophrenia that many psychiatrists prescribe for autism spectrum children and adults. The high risks associated with Risperdal are described later in this chapter. I doubt if doctors would suggest institutionalization if they knew that recovery was possible using advanced biochemical therapies. It seems clear that ABA is an excellent recommendation for families who can afford it or whose children can obtain this via the school system, and it is especially effective when used together with biochemical treatments.

Behavioral therapy

While psychotherapy and counseling have lost credibility in autism, ABA continues to be very popular and effective, and a number of different ABA protocols[130-134] are used extensively. In general, ABA involves a multitude of direct interactions with an affected child over a period of months or years. The protocols are aimed at elimination of inappropriate behaviors and development of positive behaviors to enable improvements in speech, socialization, and learning. In general, without assistance, ABA is very expensive and requires great patience. However, research studies have consistently shown benefits,[135-136] and ABA is recommended by most mainstream autism experts today. In addition to ingraining positive behaviors and traits, it's likely that ABA stimulates the development of new brain cells and synaptic connections that can result in a permanent improvement in functioning.

A good example of biomedical interventions working well together with educational/behavioral interventions exists in the area of gastrointestinal tract improvement. Many children exhibit disruptive behaviors because they are in pain from GI issues like constipation, esophageal inflammation, and reflux. A behavior plan simply won't suffice. When the underlying GI issues are addressed, such as with therapeutic diet and anti-inflammatory agents, children have less pain and exhibit behaviors more suitable to learning in a classroom. However, due to remembering the pain caused by trying to have a bowel movement, ABA behavior strategies may need to be implemented to reteach appropriate toileting habits. Repairing the gut also can accomplish the following important goals:

- Prevents undigested proteins from reaching the brain and causing aberrant behavior
- Allows desired nutrients to reach the brain and nourish it for tasks like learning
- Allows foods to be digested so that harmful overgrowths of detrimental flora (e.g., clostridia) do not proliferate, thereby releasing toxic byproducts that travel to the brain and cause detrimental behavioral effects
- Precludes further inflammation of the gut, which hithertofore would have initiated a cascade of events whereby gut inflammation increased proinflammatory immune messengers that also traveled to the brain causing immune activation

There are a multitude of biomedical therapies to choose from, with new ones introduced each year. I have arbitrarily separated them into three general categories.

General health and wellness

In many ways, children with autism are quite sick and can benefit greatly from treatments that overcome malabsorption, food sensitivities, yeast overgrowth, parasites, constipation, enuresis, poor immune function, and so on. These treatments can often provide a rapid reduction of symptoms that make life more manageable and comfortable for both the child and family. However, these treatments do not directly address the abnormalities in brain development that are central to learning, speech, and socialization.

Brain inflammation

It is increasingly clear that brain inflammation is a common feature of autism[137] that can cause irritability, erratic behavior, and diminished brain function. Treatments that reduce brain inflammation may result in striking and rapid improvements in symptoms. These benefits accrue mainly from more efficient functioning of the brain in its present state of development. As described previously, many ASD children cannot completely break down casein and gluten proteins in their diets, resulting in casomorphin and gluteomorphin aggregates[138] that can enter the brain and cause inflammation. Numerous families adopting a GF/CF diet report a rapid reduction in autism symptoms. Since brain development is a gradual process that occurs over several years, it is likely that the sudden improvements in behavior, bedwetting, speech, and socialization are due to lessening of brain inflammation.

In another example, hyperbaric therapy[139] is known to reduce brain inflammation in patients suffering from head injuries or strokes. Hyperbaric therapy has become a popular autism treatment with many reports of impressive improvements. However, in many cases, these benefits are temporary and repeated hyperbaric sessions are required to maintain improvements.

Copper overload is a distinctive feature of autism associated with inflammation, and decoppering therapies have resulted in reports of lessened autism symptoms. These are all examples of therapies that improve symptoms but may not directly enhance brain maturation. A general rule is that any autism therapy that results in sudden improvement has reduced brain inflammation but that therapy may not be the best technique for development of new brain cells, dendrites, and synaptic connections needed for advances in cognition, speech, and socialization.

Oxidative stress and damage

Recent studies indicate that severe oxidative stress is a distinctive feature of autism and may be the most important barrier to achieving proper brain function. The symptoms associated with excessive oxidative stress mirror the classic symptoms of autism spectrum disorders. If all we knew about a patient was the presence of severe oxidative stress, we would expect the following:

- Incompetent intestinal and blood-brain barriers
- Weakened immune function
- Reduced levels of digestive enzymes that break down proteins
- Tendency for yeast overload
- Depressed levels of glutathione, cysteine, and metallothionein protective proteins
- Copper overload and deficiencies of zinc and selenium
- Disruption of the one-carbon cycle resulting in undermethylation
- Reduced ability to overcome inflammation
- Hypersensitivity to mercury, lead, and other toxic metals

Each of these problems is very familiar to autism clinicians, strongly suggesting that oxidative stress is a distinctive feature of autism. Moreover, most therapies reported to benefit individuals with autism (including Risperdal) have strong antioxidant properties.

Elevated oxidative stress in the womb could modify epigenetic imprinting of gene expression, alter brain development, and weaken development of lymphoid and thymic tissues needed for immune function. Continuing oxidative stress in early childhood could alter development of brain cell minicolumns needed for learning, memory, and other cognitive functions; could inhibit brain maturation; could impair connectivity of adjacent brain regions; could increase vulnerability to toxic metals; and could alter brain neurotransmitter levels. In addition, elevated oxidative stress is associated with neurodegenerative destruction of brain cells. It appears that autism may be slowly neurodegenerative, with gradual loss of brain cells and IQ, especially after puberty. For years, I was puzzled by mainstream medicine's belief that mental retardation was common in autism, which is described in the DSM-IV-TR. After working with thousands of families, it appeared to me and my colleagues that young individuals with autism are very alert and bright, despite their odd behaviors and speech and socialization deficits. In contrast, most of our adult autism patients were heartbreaking cases involving severe mental retardation. Exceptions are Asperger's adults who generally exhibit continuing high intelligence. These observations imply that classic autism involves a tendency for gradual degeneration of brain cells and a loss of IQ. Research studies by McGinnis and colleagues[125] have indicated oxidative damage in brain tissues of children with autism. The good news is that inexpensive antioxidant therapy may overcome this tendency if continued throughout life. There are a number of antioxidant therapies including:

♦ Supplementation of glutathione, selenium, alpha lipoic acid, zinc, and vitamins C and E
♦ Methylation therapies
♦ Chelation
♦ MT-Promotion therapy (see Appendix C)

The combination of antioxidant therapy and ABA seems especially promising.

Risperdal and Brain Shrinkage: A Warning for Autism Families[140]

Risperdal is an atypical antipsychotic medication developed for schizophrenia that is often prescribed for autistic children by mainstream doctors. Published research by McCracken and others has demonstrated that this medication can effectively reduce irritability and emotional meltdowns in autistics.[141] However, the safety of Risperdal has never been established for young children, and its impact on early brain development is unknown. Recent MRI studies have heightened these concerns due to strong evidence that atypical antipsychotic medications reduce brain cortex volumes.

The first warnings came from published reports of reduced cortical gray matter volumes and glial cell numbers in macaque monkeys after administration of atypical medications.[142-144] These results were especially significant since they were very similar to the findings from postmortem studies in schizophrenia.[145] The most decisive and troubling study was published in 2011 by Beng-Chung Ho and colleagues from the University of Iowa's Department of Psychiatry.[88] The Iowa researchers studied 211 schizophrenics who underwent repeated high-resolution MRI scans over a period of 5-14 years. They found brain shrinkage similar to that observed in the monkey studies, and they also discovered that the brain volume loss was directly related to the dosage and duration of atypical medication treatment.

These results have caused great concern in the psychiatry community since atypicals have become the treatment of choice for schizophrenia patients. A February 2011 editorial[146] in the prestigious *Archives of General Psychiatry* stated that the risk/reward ratio for use of atypicals may be far greater than previously believed and urged psychiatrists to "prescribe the minimal amount(s) needed" in management of schizophrenia patients. The editorial also recommended increased use of nonpharmacological approaches and pursuit of alternate medications.

These disturbing findings do not prove that Risperdal causes brain shrinkage in children with autism since similar experiments have never been performed for this population. However, the risk of Risperdal use in young children appears very real, especially for those who have not yet completed the brain development process. Risperdal's benefits for autism patients are very real but are limited to behavioral improvements. It appears these benefits may come at an unacceptable price. The new findings of brain shrinkage after atypical medications make it very difficult to justify the use of Risperdal in autism.

The Final Battleground—the Brain

While treatments to enhance health, eliminate toxins, reduce inflammation, and overcome oxidative stress are essential, the greatest potential for progress lies in treatments aimed directly at the autistic brain. These treatment initiatives may be divided into two general categories:

*   Enhanced development of immature brain cells
*   Therapies that promote formation of new dendrites, receptors, and synaptic connections.

Brain-directed therapies may be the best way to make decisive advances in cognition, speech, and socialization, but they have received relatively little attention.

In 2000, I discovered that elevated copper and depressed zinc occurred throughout the autism spectrum, suggesting low activity of MT proteins that regulate these metals. Pervasive deficiency of ceruloplasmin (copper-binding protein) in ASD indicated that this copper elevation could not be attributed to inflammation. MT proteins are intimately involved in all phases of early brain cell development, including pruning, growth, and growth inhibition. Suspicion that low MT activity was involved in brain immaturity was supported by the fact that MT levels are highest in brain areas known to be immature in autism (e.g., amygdala, hippocampus, pineal gland, and cerebellum). Testing of ASD patients and controls revealed low MT levels in the individuals with autism. Encouraged by this knowledge, I developed an MT-Promotion therapy[147] using amino acids, minerals, and vitamins known to enhance genetic expression and regulation of MT proteins. In our patient population, this therapy resulted in clear improvements in efficacy, based on an open-label study.

Dr. Amy Holmes performed an independent study of MT-Promotion therapy and also reported excellent results. However, use of this therapy has been hindered by the proliferation of improper commercial lab tests that generated many erroneous reports of elevated MT in autism spectrum patients. A possible limitation of MT-Promotion therapy is that it doesn't directly address the reduced number of dendrites and receptors in the brain cells of persons with autism. Development of new and effective therapies to stimulate brain maturation is a very high priority. A recent discovery is the role of semaphorin proteins in guiding axonal growth to form effective synapses and minicolumns. Other promising research areas that could lead to therapies for promoting brain plasticity include parvalbumin, GABAergic signaling, and Reelin (a protein that helps regulate processes of neuronal migration and positioning). Better understanding of these processes could lead to effective therapies for improving mental functioning in autism.

A Clue from the Past—Thalidomide Babies

About 50 years ago, the world was shocked by an epidemic of physically deformed babies caused by Thalidomide, an anti-nausea pill used by many expectant mothers. Along with severe physical abnormalities, a surprisingly high number of these children developed classic autism. Researchers eventually discovered an interesting fact—autism was present only if the mother took Thalidomide between days 20-24 of gestation.[148] Since the medication was taken by thousands of mothers at different stages of their pregnancy, this window of time clearly was a period of heightened autism susceptibility. The researchers theorized that the toxic chemical interfered with closing of the neural tube, a major event occurring at this stage of embryonic development.

Another major event during days 20-24 is the establishment of many epigenetic bookmarks that determine expression rates for a multitude of genes. These marks usually are permanent, persisting throughout the life of the child. Exposure to toxic chemicals during this period can cause permanent abnormalities in physical health and mental function. An unfortunate fact is that these predispositions for autism are imprinted before most mothers know they are pregnant. The most important protective measures against autism may be those taken prior to knowledge of conception.

A handful of natural biochemical factors are dominant in epigenetic processes, with methylation and acetylation having special prominence. It is interesting to note that more than 95% of autistic children are undermethylated, and this may be central to the autism condition. After meeting thousands of affected families, I have been struck by the high percentage of competent parents who make a scientific study of autism and dedicate their entire lives to helping their children. After evaluating more than 30,000 persons for methyl status, I am convinced that most parents of autistic children exhibit symptoms of undermethylation, including high accomplishment, obsessive-compulsive traits, attention to detail, and seasonal allergies. If both parents possess the same methylation imbalance, epigenetic abnormalities are far more likely.

There is mounting evidence[149] that certain gene expression tendencies can be transmitted to future generations by the process we identified earlier as TEI. More than 100 transgenerational epigenetic conditions have been identified in early research, and many more are anticipated. Animal research has provided strong evidence of TEI, and there are early indications of TEI in humans. It is possible that TEI is a major factor in the autism epidemic. Toxic insults during days 20-24 of gestation could transfer autism predisposition to future generations, especially to nonaffected females less prone to developing autism. In this way, the population of parents at risk for giving birth to ASD children could greatly increase over time—without changes in DNA.

Bringing It All Together: An Epigenetic Model of Autism

Many of the mysteries regarding autism have been resolved, and this devastating disorder is gradually coming into clear view. I believe an important first step is to recognize that autism is a gene programming (epigenetic) disorder. Evidence of autism's epigenetic nature includes:

+ Abnormal methylation, the most decisive factor in epigenetic disorders
+ Severe oxidative overload, a condition that can produce deviant gene marks
+ Vulnerability to toxic metals and other environmental insults
+ Many cases of sudden onset after a period of relative wellness
+ Persistence of autism after onset, indicating that a life-changing event has occurred
+ Violation of classic laws of genetics in autism, a condition with a strong heritable component

It appears the combination of undermethylation, oxidative overload, and epigenetics represents the Bermuda Triangle of autism. I believe an unfortunate convergence of these three factors is the cause of most cases of autism. In essence, autism appears to be a gene programming disorder that develops in undermethyated persons who experience environmental insults that produce overwhelming oxidative stress.

In the history of science, progress has often been hastened by the development of theories that attempt to explain the mechanisms of poorly understood phenomena. In this spirit, I present the Walsh Model of Autism that is largely based on the research advances and dedicated efforts of others.

1. Predisposition to autism results from in utero hypomethylation that that causes over-expression of several genes, weakened protection against oxidative stresses, and increased vulnerability to environmental insults.

2. Sometime between conception and age three, environmental insults reach a threshold in which oxidative stresses overwhelm oxidative protectors (a tipping point). This triggers an epigenetic event in which DNA and histone marks are altered, producing the syndrome with the diagnostic label of autism. Since the deviant marks are maintained during future cell divisions, the condition doesn't go away and can result in a lifetime of disability.

3. Autism onset may occur in utero or after birth, depending on the timing and severity of the environmental insults.

4. The altered marks result in abnormal brain development, a tendency for serious brain inflammation and oxidative stress, and significant biochemical imbalances.

5. Many genes are adversely affected, producing a myriad of physical problems, such as weakened immunity, food sensitivities, seizure tendencies, heightened sensitivity to toxins, and poor behavioral control.

The Aftermath of Autism and Treatment Opportunities

Since autism involves deviant gene marks that survive many cell divisions, the condition can persist throughout life. The severity of autism may depend on the relative progress in brain development prior to inundation by oxidative stress and the number and type of deviant gene marks. With these insights, I believe the following three approaches have the highest promise for achieving major improvements in cognition, speech, and behavior.

1. *Antioxidant therapies:* Many symptoms of autism are directly related to elevated oxidative stress. The following are examples of benefits that may be achieved by effective antioxidant therapy:

   - Reduction of brain inflammation may reduce irritability and enhance development of speech, cognition, and socialization.
   - Improved glutathione and metallothionein levels can enhance memory by increasing glutamate activity at NMDA receptors.

- Reductions in the number of oxidative free radicals would enhance immune response, protein digestion, and eliminate the tendency for yeast overload.
- The filtering action of intestinal and blood-brain barriers can be improved by eliminating oxidative overload.
- Increased activity of metallothionein proteins could promote development of new brain cells and synaptic connections.
- Elimination of oxidative overloads would protect against brain cell death (apoptosis) and cognitive impairments.

It cannot be stressed enough that continuous, strong antioxidant therapy should be employed as appropriate under medical oversight in order to prevent progressive and severe cognitive deterioration as the individual with autism ages; this can be accomplished with fairly routine and inexpensive supplementation.

2. *Normalization of chromatin methyl/acetyl levels:* Undermethylation is a distinctive feature of autism that results in altered kinetics of gene expression. Epigenetic therapies aimed at increasing methyl levels at CpG islands and histone tails have great promise. In many cases, this requires removal of acetyl groups and substitution with methyl at these locations. The dominant factors that control the methyl/acetyl competition are four families of enzymes: acetylases, deacetylases, methylases, and demethylases. Standard methylation protocols may be inappropriate due to the impact of specific nutrients on these enzymes. For example, folic acid supplements can reduce chromatin methylation due to folate's powerful role in enzymatic demethylation of histones. Development of nutrient therapies to normalize methyl/acetyl levels at CpG islands and histone tails is a very fertile area for research.

3. *Reversal of deviant gene marks:* Cancer researchers are actively investigating epigenetic therapies aimed at reversing abnormal gene marks believed responsible for many types of cancer. If autism truly is an epigenetic disorder, this approach could eventually lead to effective autism prevention. For example, early infant genomic testing could determine if autism-predisposing marks are present, and it's likely that future research will identify clinical methods for normalizing the marks with natural, biochemical therapy. This line of research may represent the ultimate solution for this devastating disorder, and it should be a high national priority.

CHAPTER 8

BEHAVIORAL DISORDERS AND ADHD

Introduction

The societal problems of delinquency, crime, and violence have steadily worsened throughout our nation's history. Most of us carefully lock our doors at night for a very good reason. The USA leads the developed world in per capita rates of murder, assault, rape, and other violent crimes. We spend billions of dollars each year on law enforcement and the criminal justice system and have the world's largest prison population. Approximately 1 in every 31 American adults is in prison, on parole, or on probation. Funds badly needed for education and health care are diverted to prison construction projects. Despite the great public sacrifice, progress seems to occur at the speed of glaciers—inches per century. Our nation's report card for this subject should read: A for effort, F for accomplishment.

The basic problem is two-fold. First of all, we do not understand why some children become violent criminals and others do not. Secondly, we don't know how to reform or rehabilitate these persons once they start breaking the law. For more than a century, progress has been blocked by the belief that violent criminals are created by flawed life circumstances, such as poverty, child abuse, bad parenting, and broken homes. The reality is that most children with terrible behavior were born with chemical imbalances that predispose them to this conduct. Flawed life circumstances can aggravate this condition, but the underlying cause is usually bad brain chemistry. The best way to reduce crime and violence is to identify children with antisocial tendencies and to provide effective treatment before their lives are ruined. Until this capability is achieved, children with behavioral disorders will continue to develop into criminals, and our nation's horrific rate of crime and violence will persist.

For centuries, psychiatry has debated the relative importance of nature and nurture. During the first half of the 20th century, the social and emotional environment in childhood was considered dominant in forming a person's traits, personality, and mental health. Since then, inherited differences in brain chemistry have been identified as major factors in depression, schizophrenia, and other disorders. It is now clear that nature and nurture collaborate in the formation of a human being. A recipe for a criminal is imbalanced brain chemistry plus a bad environment.

Lessons from Prison

In the early 1970s, I organized a volunteer program at Stateville Correctional Center, a maximum security prison near Joliet, Illinois. Over the next 20 years, my group was closely associated with hundreds of persons who had committed violent crimes. Initially, we developed recreation programs and assisted inmates who were being brutalized or who were seriously ill. We learned that prison is a revolving door with most parolees returning to a life of crime. Many are career criminals or gang members who have no desire to reform. Others sincerely intend to be law-abiding but usually fail. We learned that many parolees are shunned by their families and potential employers. It's a danger to society for these persons to become hungry and homeless since they know illegal ways to make money quickly. In 1974, with the goal of crime prevention, I organized an ex-offender program to help ex-convicts integrate into society. This activity brought me into close contact with dozens of families who had produced a criminal. This was the beginning of my education regarding the causes of behavioral disorders.

A high percentage of the ex-convicts were from broken homes and deprived neighborhoods. However, a surprising number were raised in a good environment along with brothers and sisters who had become productive law-abiding citizens. Several parents said their wayward children seemed different from birth and resisted their attempts at love and nurturing. They spoke of children who started to lie as soon as they learned to talk, became assaultive by age three, tortured family pets, and were oppositional and defiant by age four. Many future criminals had counseling and psychotherapy before kindergarten, psychiatric medications by age six, hospitalization by age nine, and incarceration by age 12. The families reported that physical punishment was completely ineffective as was behavior modification and counseling. I met two desperate families who believed their child was possessed and had tried exorcism. I learned that the parent of a criminal is often a parent with a broken heart.

About 50% of my volunteers were colleagues at Argonne National Laboratory, and we began to question the prevailing belief that criminals are created by adverse life experiences. At this time, depression and schizophrenia were known to have an inherited component involving disordered brain chemistry. We started collecting samples of blood, urine, and tissues from prisoners and ex-convicts for chemical analysis. Our initial tests involved persons with a history of extreme violence, including several refugees from death row. For nearly 12 months, our results were inconclusive with no biochemical differences observed between criminals and nonviolent controls. Our first success was the discovery in 1974 of distinctive trace metal imbalances in the violent group. Encouraged by this finding, we studied metal levels in hundreds of prisoners, ex-convicts, and violent children in the Chicago area. We consistently found abnormal levels of copper, zinc, lead, cadmium, chromium, manganese, calcium, magnesium, sodium, potassium, lithium, and cobalt in the blood, urine, and hair of persons with behavioral disorders. With the approval of Argonne management, I organized a formal experiment to compare trace metal concentrations in violent persons and well-behaved controls. Argonne's resident epidemiologist, Dr. Robert Lundy, recommended a sibling study to minimize environmental differences in the two groups. Argonne's Ken Jensen developed analytical chemistry techniques to ensure valid metal assays. I then spent eight months searching for families with a violent son and a well-behaved brother in the same household.

Sibling experiment

Our test group consisted of 24 pairs of brothers who lived in the same household and attended the same school. Each pair consisted of a child with a history of delinquency and violent assaults and a brother with ideal behavior and good academics. In essence, we found 24 families with a proverbial child from hell and an all-American boy living in the same family. The age range was 8 to 18 years for both groups with a median age of 15 years. The samples were coded and blinded to the testing laboratory and the researchers.

After breaking the code, we learned that most of the well-behaved controls had the expected levels of the trace metals tested. In contrast, most violent subjects exhibited abnormal levels, especially with respect to copper, zinc, lead, and cadmium. In general, the violent children exhibited higher lead and cadmium levels than did the controls. However, this test group was about evenly split between children with elevated Cu/Zn ratios and others with depressed Cu/Zn ratios. None of the well-behaved children exhibited a Cu/Zn imbalance. We used a parent questionnaire to determine if there were significant behavioral differences between the two violent cohorts. The results of the survey were exciting and provocative. Most parents of high Cu/Zn children reported "Jekyll-Hyde" behavior, with periods of very good behavior interrupted by violent episodes. Most reported genuine remorse after the meltdowns. The children with low Cu/Zn ratios presented a very different picture. Most were described as oppositional, defiant, assaultive, cruel to animals, with several families reporting fascination with fire. This latter group clearly fit the psychiatric definition of antisocial personality disorder.[73] In contrast, the high Cu/Zn group had symptoms associated with intermittent explosive disorder. This experiment yielded clear evidence of trace metal abnormalities in males with behavioral disorders. A limitation of these findings was that two different behavioral biotypes had not been expected or hypothesized. My colleagues and I decided another experiment was needed, this time with many more subjects and a hypothesis of Cu/Zn imbalances in the violent group.

Field test

The second formal experiment began in 1976. It involved 96 extremely violent males and 96 nonviolent male controls from the Chicago area. The two groups were matched by age, race, and socioeconomic status. In each group, one-third were African-Americans, one-third Hispanics, and one-third of European descent. The test population was composed of prison residents, ex-convicts, first offenders, and juveniles with a history of extreme violence. Half of the violent subjects were incarcerated with the remaining 50% living in society. This controlled for artifacts of prison environment, such as diet and high stress, which could blur the data.

As in the sibling study, the samples were blinded to the testing laboratory and the researchers. Upon breaking the code, we learned that 35 violent subjects exhibited elevated Cu/Zn ratios, 57 had low Cu/Zn, with the remaining four testing with normal copper and zinc. Three nonviolent controls had abnormal Cu/Zn ratios, and 93 did not. The results confirmed the findings of the sibling experiment. We now had solid evidence that abnormal copper and zinc levels were associated with violent behavior.

The results of the sibling study and field test were presented at an annual meeting of the American Criminology Association and were featured in a cover story in *Science News* magazine. The Violence Research Foundation funded two studies in which coded samples from California prison and jail residents were mingled with samples from nonviolent controls. In both cases, we were successful in identifying the criminals with better than 90% accuracy based on chemistry alone. However, two important questions were still unanswered:

- What other biochemical imbalances are associated with criminality?
- Could medical treatment of the imbalances improve behavior and enable reduced crime rates?

Collaboration with Carl Pfeiffer

The eminent Dr. Carl Pfeiffer became interested in our research and agreed to test violent criminals at his center in Princeton, New Jersey, beginning in 1976. His first subjects were five ex-convicts believed to be sociopaths who tested with low Cu/Zn ratios. Pfeiffer found each to have a curious combination of elevated blood histamine, elevated urine pyrroles, zinc deficiency, low-normal serum copper, and low blood spermine (a natural biochemical involved in cell metabolism). Over the next 12 years, Pfeiffer assisted in the evaluation of more than 500 persons with behavioral disorders. Based on chemical testing and diagnosis of chemistry imbalances, Pfeiffer prescribed treatments using amino acids, minerals, and vitamins aimed at normalizing chemistry. We soon learned that most adult criminals were prone to noncompliance and failed to achieve long-term improvements. However, this therapy brought consistent reports of great benefits from parents of violent children. In an early open-label outcome study of 100 children, two-thirds of the families reported that violent episodes and destruction of property had either ceased or become less frequent.

About 50% of the children treated by Dr. Pfeiffer for a behavioral disorder also were diagnosed with a learning disability or ADHD, and many families reported major improvements in academics following treatment. In 1986, we began treatment of well-behaved children diagnosed with ADHD with similar success. These positive results led to the 1989 founding of the Pfeiffer Treatment Center, a nonprofit clinic in Illinois specializing in patients with behavioral or learning disorders.

Biochemistry of Behavioral Disorders and ADHD

Over the past 35 years, I've collected a massive database of 1.5 million chemical assays from testing of 10,000 patients with behavioral disorders and 5,600 patients with ADHD. The data reveal a high incidence of chemical abnormalities for both groups, especially disorders of metal metabolism, methylation, pyrroles, toxic metals, glucose, and absorption. All of these imbalances have known impacts on brain functioning. As described in Chapter 3, copper is an important factor in the conversion of dopamine to norepinephrine; zinc is needed for efficient regulation of GABA; vitamin B-6 is a cofactor in the synthesis of several neurotransmitters; methionine and folic acid have powerful impacts on synaptic activity; and toxic overloads can impair brain function. Our database clearly shows that nutrient imbalances are a distinctive feature of behavioral disorders and ADHD.

Significant chemical imbalances were found in 94% of the 10,000 persons in my behavior database. Many of the remaining 6% had a history of a serious head injury, epilepsy, or oxygen deprivation during birth. The incidence of chemical imbalances for the ADHD population was about 86%. Males outnumbered females by a three-to-one ratio in both groups. The vast database revealed strong correlations between chemical abnormalities and specific behavioral disorders and ADHD:

* *Intermittant explosive disorder (IED):* My chemistry database contains more than 1,500 children who were generally well-behaved and cooperative except for occasional explosions of uncontrollable rage. Some parents referred to this behavior as an erupting volcano or a runaway train. In most cases, the episode would end within 15-30 minutes, and the child would have remorse and might beg forgiveness. However, the meltdowns would continue and often involved physical assaults and destruction of property. About 90% of IED children exhibit a very elevated Cu/Zn ratio in blood, often coincident with elevated urine pyrroles. Most families report somewhat improved behavior during the first week of nutrient therapy, with about 60 days needed for the full effect. Any ongoing psychiatric medications are continued during the first two to three months of nutrient therapy, with about 80% of the families reporting success in weaning the child off the drugs without a return of the explosions.

* *Oppositional-defiant disorder (ODD):* Many parents described their child as having a will of iron with opposition to all authority figures since age two. Typically they were described as overly stubborn, rebellious, controlling, and argumentative with adults. Several families said that simply saying the word "no" could start World War III. ODD children usually have problems making friends since they always insist on calling the shots. Academic performance is highly erratic, often depending on whether they like or dislike the teacher. About half of ODD children have a history of physical assaults, while the others restrict themselves to verbal outbursts. The classic chemical signature of ODD is undermethylation, which can be identified using blood tests for SAMe/SAH ratio, histamine, absolute basophils, etc. This imbalance is associated with low activity of dopamine and serotonin neurotransmitters. Psychiatric drugs for ODD usually involve stimulants (Ritalin, etc.) or antidepressants aimed at increasing activity of these neurotransmitters. My colleagues and I developed a nutrient therapy approach for ODD involving supplements of methionine and SAMe, while avoiding folates and choline. This nutrient protocol has two aims:

  - Increasing serotonin and dopamine levels in the brain
  - Suppressing formation of transporters at synapses

A high percentage of successfully treated patients have been able to eliminate psychiatric medications without a return of the bad behavior. A major barrier to success is the innate tendency of undermethylated patients to be noncompliant with any treatment.

- *Conduct disorder (CD):* Conduct disorder is a behavioral and emotional disorder that is present in approximately 9% of boys and 2% of girls under the age of 18. Children with conduct disorder act out aggressively and express anger inappropriately. They engage in a variety of antisocial and destructive acts, including violence toward people and animals, destruction of property, lying, stealing, truancy, and running away from home. In early childhood, many become bullies and enjoy getting into fights. They are prone to abusing drugs and alcohol and having sex at an early age. Irritability, temper tantrums, and low self-esteem are common personality traits of children with CD, and many are also oppositional and defiant. The classic chemical signature of CD is a combination of severe pyrrole disorder and undermethylation.

- *Antisocial personality disorder (ASPD):* Persons with this condition are sometimes referred to as sociopaths or psychopaths. Early warning signs include bedwetting, cruelty to animals, and fascination with fire. In most cases, they are oppositional and defiant by age 4 and exhibit a conduct disorder by age 10. Many go on to a life of crime and violence. In my 18 years as a prison volunteer, I was closely associated with more than 200 persons with this diagnosis and observed the following general characteristics:

  - Extreme narcissism – total absence of care and concern for others
  - Engaging personality and good verbal skills
  - Hypersexuality
  - Easily enraged, especially after consuming alcohol
  - High pain threshold
  - Disregard for laws and social norms
  - Fearless use of illegal drugs
  - Low opinion of normal people, who they believe are cowards
  - Impulsive actions without regard for consequences

The chemical signature of ASPD is an odd combination of undermethylation, pyrrole disorder, elevated toxic metals, severe zinc deficiency, and low-normal copper levels. Nutrient therapy to correct these imbalances generally results in reports of great improvement in ASPD children, but there is little sustainable benefit for teens or adults actively abusing alcohol or illegal drugs. This condition is treatable, but early intervention is essential.

♦ *Nonviolent behavioral disorders:* My chemistry database includes more than 1,000 persons with serious behavioral disorders who have no history of physical violence. Most cases involved poor academics and work performance along with a tendency for lying, stealing, and deceptive practices. Outcome studies indicate these persons respond well to nutrient therapy. Chemical studies indicate that most patients with a nonviolent behavioral disorder fit into one of the following biochemical classifications:

- Malabsorbers who exhibit low levels of most vitamins, minerals and amino acids
- Persons with severe glucose dyscontrol
- Nonviolent, undermethylated persons with ODD

Biochemistry of ADHD

Attention deficit hyperactivity disorder is an umbrella term given to several different learning disorders. My chemical database of 5,600 ADHD cases indicates that 75% of these persons also have a history of a significant behavioral disorder. There are three major subtypes of ADHD,[73] and each has a different chemical signature:

1. *Predominantly inattentive:* These persons may have normal or high intelligence but exhibit poor focus and concentration. They are often described as space cadets. In school, they may sit quietly, but they have little interest in the subject matter and are prone to daydreaming. Many of these children have excellent behavioral control and socialization but very poor academics. More than half of these persons are deficient in folic acid, vitamin B-12, zinc, and choline, and they develop better focus after supplements of these nutrients. Another cause of inattention can be extreme boredom, especially in children of very high intelligence, and these children need to be intellectually challenged.

2. *Predominantly impulsive and hyperactive:* These persons tend to be in constant motion, are highly distractible, and have a short attention span. As a result, they underachieve academically, regardless of their intelligence level. The classic chemical signature for this group is a metal metabolism disorder involving copper overload and zinc deficiency. As described in Chapter 3, this metal imbalance is associated with low dopamine and elevated norepinephrine and adrenalin activity. Ritalin, Adderal, and other stimulant medications can effectively elevate dopamine activity and improve academics. However, nutrient

therapy to balance copper and zinc levels can often achieve the same result without the unpleasant side effects[107] associated with stimulant medications, including appetite suppression, delayed growth, tic disorders, and personality change. It is interesting to note that Ritalin and cocaine share the same mechanism of action—dopamine reuptake inhibition by impairing the action of DAT transport proteins. Cocaine provides a sudden high due to rapid elevation of dopamine activity and is highly addictive. Ritalin taken orally causes a much slower dopamine activity rise and is generally not addictive.

3. *Combined hyperactive/impulsive and inattentive:* This largest subtype of ADHD generally involves more severe academic underachievement than subtypes 1 and 2. This population includes persons with more than one chemical imbalance, and lab testing is essential to successful diagnosis and treatment. About 68% exhibit a seriously elevated Cu/Zn ratio in blood and tissues, and normalization of these trace metals can greatly reduce hyperactivity and improve attention span. Others in this classification may have a methylation disorder, toxic overload, pyrrole disorder, or other imbalance, and blood and urine testing is necessary for accurate diagnosis.

Longitudinal studies indicate that a person's biochemical tendencies persist throughout life, suggesting they are genetic or epigenetic in origin. In many cases, symptoms of a particular imbalance have been clearly evident since infancy. The impact on a person's life depends on the severity of the chemical imbalance and environmental factors. For example, a child with a mild tendency for aggressive behavior or ADHD may develop normally if there is a good diet, an absence of serious traumatic events, and a nurturing family. However, a child born with the severe chemistry we observed in serial killers is likely to become a criminal unless the brain chemistry is corrected. Counseling and a good environment may be effective in mild-to-moderate behavioral disorders or ADHD, but our words from Chapter 3 bear repeating: a severe chemical imbalance cannot be loved away, and treatment must focus on correcting brain chemistry. Similarly, a mild genetic tendency for depression may be overcome by a good environment and counseling, whereas a severe tendency may require aggressive biochemical intervention. All of these patients are good candidates for individualized nutrient therapy.

For decades, environmental factors have been accepted as the root cause of aberrant behavior. Our research indicates that imbalanced brain chemistry is equally important. For many humans, the recipe for bad behavior is biochemical predisposition plus a flawed environment.

Nutrient Therapy Outcomes

It is sometimes difficult for doctors to determine the effectiveness of novel treatments, especially in medical practices that involve infrequent return visits. Five or ten percent of patients may send letters of gratitude that report great progress. However, an important question is "What happened to the other 90-95 percent?" Most therapies entail a significant placebo effect, and ineffective treatments will invariably generate sincere reports of improvement due to this. An effective solution is to occasionally spot-check results by contacting a large number of consecutive patients and determining the overall outcomes.

Since 1976, I've conducted more than a dozen outcome studies to measure effectiveness of nutrient therapy for BD and ADHD patients. The early studies

---

Table 8-1.
Early Behavior Findings: 1978-1988

- About 65% of families reported improved behavior, with better results for young children.

- About 80% of children under age 14 exhibited improved behavior, with more than half ceasing physical violence altogether.

- A gradual decline in efficacy was observed after age 14.

- Higher efficacy was reported for severe cases involving a history of frequent assaultive behavior.

- Most persons diagnosed with oppositional-defiant disorder were undermethylated.

- Most persons diagnosed with conduct disorder had elevated urine pyrroles.

- About two-thirds of ADHD children exhibited an elevated Cu/Zn ratio in blood.

- Many families reported compliance problems, with more than 10% failing to initiate treatment.

- About 15% reported occasional nausea or stomach pain if nutrients were taken on an empty stomach.

---

involved hundreds of consecutive patients who received nutrient therapy, and they provided information on treatment success rates, side effects, and compliance problems. Some of the early lessons learned are summarized in Table 8-1. An important finding was that the treatments appeared to be highly effective for young children, with a steady decline in efficacy after age 14. Most patients abusing cocaine or other illegal substances had zero detectible progress. Excessive alcohol intake also correlated with absence of progress. Another explanation for poorer results with adults was that the years of bad behavior may have fostered an ingrained negative self-image. By 1985, our emphasis changed from adult criminals to children with behavioral disorders.

All of the early outcome studies indicated significant compliance problems attributed to the number and taste of capsules. In 2003, we developed a compounding pharmacy to reduce the capsules by a factor of two to three. In addition, we learned that tiny amounts of vanillin and other neutral substances could mask the disagreeable taste and increase compliance rates.

The early outcome studies also revealed that treatment success rates improved when we adopted a primary nurse system in which each patient was assigned a staff nurse responsible for assisting the family in understanding the treatment approach and overcoming compliance problems.

Year 2004 Outcome Study

In 2004, we published an open-label outcome study[150] that measured the effectiveness of our nutrient therapy system for 207 patients with behavioral disorders. The clinical procedure included a medical history, lab assays of 90 biochemical factors, and a physical exam. Standardized treatment protocols were applied for each imbalance that was identified. The frequencies of physical assaults and destructive episodes were determined before and after treatment, with follow-up ranging from four to eight months.

Each of the 207 test subjects had a prior diagnosis of conduct disorder, oppositional-defiant disorder, antisocial personality disorder, or ADHD. The test population was comprised of 149 males and 58 females, and most had a history of extreme violence. More than 95% had received behavior modification, conflict resolution, counseling, and/or psychotherapy prior to seeking nutrient therapy, and 85% had a history of Ritalin, antidepressants, or other psychiatric medications. In all cases, serious behavioral problems were still evident. The most common chemical imbalances and the therapies prescribed are described below.

Elevated copper/zinc ratio: A total of 75.4% of test subjects exhibited elevated serum copper and depressed plasma zinc. Behavioral disorders associated with this imbalance include episodic rage disorder, attention-deficit disorder, and hyperactivity. Treatment involved MT promotion therapy using zinc, glutathione, selenium, and cysteine together with augmenting nutrients such as pyridoxine, ascorbic acid, and vitamin E.

Overmethylation: About 29.5% of the BD subjects exhibited depressed blood histamine, which is a biomarker for overmethylation, an elevated methyl/folate ratio, and elevated levels of dopamine and norepinephrine. This imbalance is associated with anxiety, paranoia, and depression and was treated using folic acid, vitamins B-3 and B-12, and augmenting nutrients.

Undermethylation: A total of 37.7% of the patients exhibited elevated blood histamine, a biomarker for undermethylation and a depressed methyl/folate ratio. This imbalance is associated with depression, seasonal allergies, obsessive-compulsive tendencies, high libido, and low levels of serotonin. Treatment involved supplements of methionine, calcium, magnesium, and vitamins B-6, C, and D.

Pyrrole disorder: This imbalance was exhibited by 32.9% of the patients. Elevated pyrroles have been associated with an inborn error of pyrrole chemistry, but this also can result from porphyria or exposure to heavy metals, toxic chemicals, and other conditions enhancing oxidative stress. This imbalance results in severe deficiencies of pyridoxine and zinc and is associated with poor stress control and explosive anger. Treatment for this disorder involved supplements of pyridoxine, pyridoxal-5-phosphate, zinc, and vitamins C and E.

Heavy metal overload: Elevated levels of lead, cadmium, or other toxic metals were exhibited by 17.9% of the BD persons. Toxic metal overloads have been associated with behavioral disorders and academic underachievement. Treatment involved supplementation with calcium, zinc, manganese, pyridoxine, selenium, and other antioxidants to promote the excretion of toxic metals.

Glucose dyscontrol: Among the test population, 30.4% exhibited a tendency for unusually low blood glucose levels. This imbalance appears to represent an aggravating factor rather than a cause of behavioral disorders. Treatment involved supplements of chromium picolinate and manganese along with dietary modifications.

Malabsorption: A total of 15.5% exhibited a malabsorption syndrome involving generalized low levels of amino acids, vitamins, and minerals. This chemical imbalance has been associated with irritability, impulsivity, and underachievement. Treatment varied, depending on the type of malabsorption (for example, low stomach acid, gastric insufficiency, yeast overgrowth, or a brush border disorder). The treatments included the use of nutrients for regulating stomach acid levels, digestive enzymes, biotin, and probiotics.

Treatment effectiveness results: Compliance is a major barrier to treatment success in behavioral disorders. For example, it is very difficult to get an oppositional-defiant teenager to do anything, including swallowing a number of capsules daily. In this study of 207 subjects, a total of 76% remained compliant at the time of the follow-up interview. The families reported that about 50% of the noncompliant persons never began treatment. The behavioral improvements achieved in the compliant group are summarized in Figures 8-1 and 8-2.

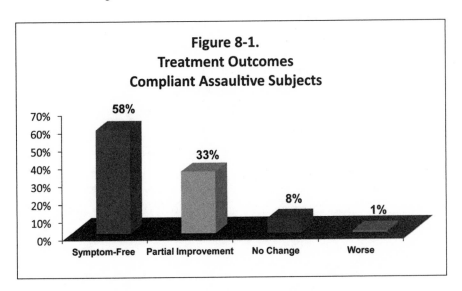

A total of 91% of families reported a reduced incidence of physical assaults, with 58% reporting that assaults had completely stopped. Similar results were obtained with respect to destruction of property (Figure 8-2). These results clearly indicate that individualized nutrient therapy had been effective in improving behaviors. Statistical significance (p<0.001) was found both for reduced frequency of assaults and destructive incidents, indicating less than one chance in a thousand that the improvements were not related to the nutrient therapy. Treatment effectiveness was highest for children under the age of 14. This finding may be due to the reduced incidence of serious drug/alcohol abuse and a less ingrained negative self-image in this younger population.

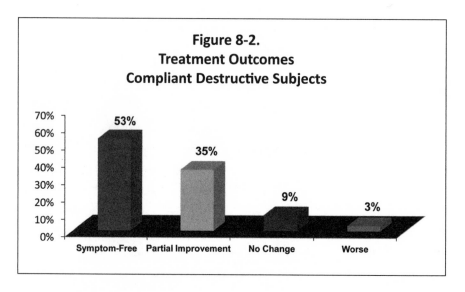

Inner City School Project

Free medical testing and nutrient therapy were provided to 33 at-risk children attending a K-8 school in a high poverty Chicago neighborhood. The ages ranged from 5 to 14 years, and most had a prior diagnosis of severe ADHD or a BD. Participating students were selected by the school's special education staff, who also evaluated their academic and behavioral status before and after treatment. The protocol included a medical history, physical examination by a physician, and extensive lab testing. The medical procedures were streamlined, and the total cost was reduced to $300/child. The inner city parents were very dedicated to helping their troubled children, and only three failed to achieve compliance. This two-year program was funded by the National Recreation Foundation.

ADHD students: Fourteen ADHD children were evaluated before and after treatment, based on the Iowa Tests of Basic Skills testing and teacher reports. A total of 71% achieved a significant improvement in academics according to the special education staff. Some of the improvements were quite spectacular. A nine-year-old female improved her Iowa Tests reading score from the 13th percentile to the 71st percentile after six months of treatment. Her math scores improved from the 36th percentile to the 51st percentile, and staff and parents described her as "emerging from her shell." In another example, a seven-year-old girl became calmer and more focused and had a striking improvement on the Iowa Tests reading and math batteries. Four of the ADHD students failed to exhibit academic improvement.

BD students: The special education staff reported that 13 out of the 16 students with serious behavioral problems had improved. There were several cases in which reports of serious assaultive behavior completely stopped. A 13-year-old who had been suspended several times for out-of-control behavior became calm, and his explosive anger completely ceased. In addition, he was able to maintain good behavior after discontinuing Ritalin. A six-year-old who was actively engaged in hitting and kicking fellow students completely stopped his violent actions. Several parents said they had feared their child was heading for prison and were now thrilled with the improvement. In general, the behavioral improvements for these inner city youths were better than we have achieved for children living in wealthy suburbs or rural areas. Society has known for decades that inner city high poverty areas are a breeding ground for crime. This project's results suggest that individualized nutrient therapy provided to at-risk, inner city children may be an effective crime prevention strategy.

Nutrient Therapy Timeframes

The time required for academic improvement is generally longer than that for behavioral improvements. Correction of chemical imbalances does not inject new knowledge into a child's brain, but it can greatly increase the rate of learning. In both cases, the timing of progress depends on the individual imbalances that are treated. The most rapid progress is achieved by pyrrole disorder patients who may become calmer after a few days of therapy. The slowest imbalance to resolve is undermethylation, with 30-60 days typically required before improvements are observed. Three factors can delay progress:

- Type A blood
- Malabsorption
- Hypoglycemia

Some unfortunate patients have all three factors and require six months of treatment before success is achieved. Nutrient therapy for ADHD children usually requires three months to achieve full effect. ADHD adults respond more slowly, with more than six months often required before progress begins. BD patients usually respond to nutrient therapy within two weeks, with full effect achieved after two months. Our outcome studies have consistently shown that children with behavioral disorders achieve the most rapid improvements and highest efficacy rates of all patient groups.

Epigenetics and Crime Prevention

A high percentage of serious crimes are committed by persons diagnosed with antisocial personality disorder, previously referred to as sociopaths. This group includes nearly all serial killers and serial rapists as well as numerous career criminals. Other persons who cause great societal harm are pedophiles and other persons with certain forms of perverted sexuality such as necrophilia. As described in Chapter 4, my extensive database indicates that both of these criminal classifications fit the criteria for an epigenetic disorder. This suggests that epigenetics research has potential to identify the gene expression errors associated with these criminal behaviors. In this event, children could be screened with blood testing soon after birth, and epigenetic therapies could be developed to eliminate these severe behavioral disorders. This may represent the world's most promising approach for crime prevention and would provide great benefits to these children and their families. Epigenetics research studying criminal behavior should be a high national priority.

For decades, researchers have debated the relative influence of nature and nurture[151] in rage disorders, crime, violence, etc. The high incidence of biochemical imbalances in populations with behavioral disorders and the major behavioral improvements following correction of imbalances strongly suggests that biochemistry has a powerful influence on human behavior. Effective prevention of delinquency and crime may require early intervention aimed at normalizing the brain chemistry of at-risk children. Assessment of this therapy as a crime prevention measure will require the following:

+ Double-blind, placebo-controlled studies to decisively measure treatment efficacy
+ Longitudinal studies to determine if the behavioral improvements seen after four to eight months of therapy are enduring

The relatively inexpensive intervention of nutrient therapy can reduce crime and violence, reduce human suffering, and save billions of dollars annually.

CHAPTER 9

ALZHEIMER'S DISEASE

Introduction

In 1905, German psychiatrist Alois Alzheimer performed an autopsy on a woman who had suffered an early cognitive decline. He discovered that about one-third of the woman's cortical brain cells had deteriorated, leaving a plaque (an extracellular protein buildup) and tangled cell fragments. Similar findings had been reported earlier by other researchers, but Alzheimer provided a much more detailed and accurate description of the diseased brain.[152] At the time, Alzheimer was working at the laboratory of Emil Kraepelin, the renowned discoverer of manic depression (now known as bipolar disorder) and the leading psychiatrist of his time. In 1910, Kraepelin published a *Handbook of Psychiatry*[153] in which he referred to this form of dementia as Alzheimer's disease in honor of his friend and colleague.

More than 100 years have passed, and Alzheimer's disease (AD) is still poorly understood and generally regarded as incurable. AD is a progressive, fatal brain disease affecting about 4.5 million Americans. The first signs are reduced sense of smell and inability to retain short-term memories. As the relentless destruction of brain cells proceeds, the ability to function declines drastically. Aricept and other medications can enable the deteriorating brain to perform better for 4-12 months, but they fail to stop the rate of cell destruction. The average time between diagnosis and death is about seven years. Many AD patients attempt to disguise their symptoms in the early stages. In 2007, we evaluated an old friend who called me by name and carried on a brief conversation that didn't betray his AD condition. His wife had reminded him of my name a few seconds before our meeting, but testing revealed that he thought Harry Truman was still president. AD is a disease feared by most senior citizens for good reason. About one-third of the population is in some stage of AD by the time they reach the age of 85. The latter stages are especially difficult as the patient no longer recognizes loved ones and may experience depression, anxiety, irritability, and declining physical health.

Stages of Alzheimer's Disease

1. *Early warning signs:* Many patients exhibit subtle symptoms of AD several years prior to diagnosis. The most common indications are loss of interest in events and activities along with a decline in mental sharpness. This condition is often called mild cognitive impairment.

2. *Mild Alzheimer's disease:* A formal diagnosis of AD usually is made when there is a striking loss of recent memories, while older memories are still retained. Another diagnostic symptom is a shrinking vocabulary and loss of communication skills. The popular mini-mental state examination (MMSE) test[154] is helpful in establishing a diagnosis; it is based on a patient's ability to perform simple tasks such as counting backward from 100 by threes or copying a drawing of a pentagon. A more decisive test is the computerized CANTAB Test[155] (Cambridge Neuropsychological Test Automated Battery). In this stage of the disease, most persons still enjoy life and can accomplish basic tasks but require supervision for activities requiring complex thought or logic.

3. *Moderate Alzheimer's disease:* The deterioration of neurons eventually spreads throughout the brain and the patient loses the ability to perform many common activities of daily living. Memory continues to deteriorate, and the patient may no longer recognize his own grandchildren or recent friends. Reading and writing skills gradually disappear, and irritability, wandering, falling, and physical aggression symptoms can be very challenging for the family. About one-third of AD victims develop delusions and urinary incontinence. Most families are forced to move their loved one to a long-term care facility when they can no longer cope with the worsening symptoms. While heartbreaking for the family, this step frequently does not seem to bother the patient.

4. *Advanced Alzheimer's disease:* During this final stage, the patient becomes completely dependent on caregivers. As the disease progresses, many develop a wooden expression, lose the ability to speak, and fail to respond to visitors. In the final stages, they become bedridden, totally incontinent, and unable to feed themselves. Death usually results from an infection, respiratory problems, etc. and not directly from AD itself.[156]

The Role of Genetics

Although the cause of AD is still unknown, it is clear that genetics or epigenetics play an important role. There are two types of AD and both have genetic links. *Familial AD*[157] typically develops between the ages of 40 and 55 and represents about 5% of cases. This condition is caused by mutations to genes that produce presenilin 1, presenilin 2, or amyloid precursor protein (APP). The *late-onset* form of AD represents about 95% of cases, usually developing after age 70. In 1993, researchers at Duke University[158] reported that an apolipoprotein E (ApoE) abnormality represents a powerful risk factor in late-onset AD. ApoE is a protein containing 299 amino acids that can exist in three isoforms: E2, E3, and E4. Isoform E3 is identical to that of E2 except that a cysteine in the amino acid chain is replaced by arginine. In isoform E4, two cysteines are replaced by arginine. The risk of developing AD is lowest in ApoE2, intermediate in ApoE3, and highest in ApoE4. Persons born with an E4 allele from both parents are between 10 and 30 times more likely to develop AD by age 75 when compared with persons without an E4 allele. However, many persons with both E4 alleles live to a ripe old age without developing memory loss or other symptoms of dementia. Moreover, 40% of AD victims do not have the E4 gene. Genetic testing can determine a person's ApoE type, but it has not become popular due to the perception that the disease is incurable. The bottom line is that ApoE4 represents an AD risk factor but does not doom a person to acquiring the disease. In a positive development, several risk factors have been identified that may enable a person to reduce the likelihood of acquiring AD.

Risk Factors

The following factors increase the likelihood that a person will experience Alzheimer's disease.

- *Age:* Life expectancy was only 45-50 years in the early 1900s, and few persons lived long enough to develop AD. For many years, the connection between AD and advanced age went unnoticed. In 1960, British researchers[159] discovered that most cases of senility were actually AD, with clear evidence of amyloid plaques and tangles within brain cells. We now know that more than 90% of AD cases are diagnosed after age 70. The likelihood of this disease increases sharply with age, and about one-third of persons reaching age 85 are in some stage of the disorder. Surprisingly, there is evidence that the risk of AD declines after age 90.

- *Head injury:* Studies[160] have found a strong association between head injuries and AD. This factor is most evident in persons who have had multiple blows to the head, including boxers and football players. In 1993, the British Medical Association[161] reported evidence that boxers have an increased risk for AD, and some acquire the disorder before age 40. An example is provided by three boxers in the Quarry family who all developed serious dementia, including Jerry Quarry, who once fought for the world heavyweight championship, His family has established a foundation for AD research.

- *Education level:* In 2008, Washington University scientists[162] reported that persons with higher education levels had a lower AD risk when compared with the rest of the population. This was based on positron emission tomography (PET) scans that directly measured the amount of plaque in brains of living persons. The data indicated that persons who didn't complete grade school were four times more likely to acquire AD than college graduates. A recent study[163] has indicated that higher education delays the onset of AD but that the disease progresses more rapidly once AD has begun in these persons.

- *Mental activity:* Three studies[164] have indicated that mentally stimulating activities such as playing bridge, doing puzzles, or learning a new language reduce the risk of AD. This suggests that sitting on the couch and watching TV too regularly may be dangerous to your health.

- *Physical activity:* Persons engaging in regular physical activity[165] were found to have reduced AD risk. However, it's possible this is due to better cardiovascular health or reduced obesity rather that a direct result of physical exercise.

- *Vascular factors:* The first brain areas damaged in AD are very close to blood vessels. In addition, there is published evidence[166] that a variety of cardiovascular problems increase AD risk. Examples include strokes, hypertension, hypotension, atrial fibrillation, atherosclerosis, and elevated serum homocysteine.

- *Alcohol use:* An interesting finding is that persons who drink moderate amounts of alcohol are better protected against AD than those who never consume alcohol. In the Copenhagen Heart Study,[167] red wine was found to be especially effective. One or two glasses of red wine daily have been recommended for persons with no history of alcoholism. There is also evidence that high alcohol consumption (including red wine) increases the likelihood of AD.

- *Physical illness:* Persons with a history of diabetes or other autoimmune diseases appear to have a higher risk of AD. The strongest data[168] are for type 2 diabetes and insulin resistance.

♦ *Toxic metals:* There is some evidence[169] that aluminum, mercury, and other toxic metals are associated with AD. Mercury in particular has become a highly controversial issue. On one hand, there is published data showing a positive association between mercury exposure and the risk of AD, and this has led many persons to have their dental amalgams removed. In addition, mercury exposure causes increased oxidative stress and this factor is elevated in AD. Dental amalgams result in a significant vapor pressure of mercury, and these vapors can be directly absorbed by lung capillaries. On the other hand, other studies have reported no correlation between the number of amalgam fillings and AD, and the American Dental Association has aggressively denied any relationship between amalgams and AD. Another source of mercury for many seniors is an annual flu shot.

♦ *Poor nutrition:* Inadequate nutrition is a common problem in elderly populations, and low levels of zinc and vitamins A, C, and E result in increased oxidative stress. Several studies[170] indicate that oxidative stress plays an important role in the development of AD. In addition, elevated serum homocysteine is a known AD risk factor[171] that can result from deficiencies of folic acid and vitamin B-12. A high-quality diet may represent an important protective factor against AD.

Alzheimer's Disease Theories

1. *Cholinergic theory:* The cholinergic theory[172] was prominent in the 1980s and early 1990s and continues to be the basis for most of today's AD medications. This theory states that AD begins with the depletion of acetylcholine activity in the brain. Acetylcholine is a major neurotransmitter important for memory processes and is seriously depleted in AD brains. This has been attributed to a shortage of enzymes (choline acetyltransferase and acetylcholine esterase) necessary for production and regulation of acetylcholine. For years, these low enzyme levels were believed to cause physical problems with at-risk neurons and trigger the cell death process. However, it was eventually learned that the low enzyme levels are not present during early stages of AD but appear later. This is strong evidence[173] that the cholinergic theory of AD onset is incorrect and that the low acetylcholine and enzyme levels are an aftermath and not a cause of the disease. Aricept and other acetylcholine-enhancing medications are still widely used since they can provide temporary memory improvement for the dying patient. The bottom line is that these medications provide 4-12 months

of improved brain function, but they do little or nothing to stop the relentless destruction of the brain.

2. *Amyloid plaque hypothesis:* The theory with the largest following is the amyloid hypothesis[174-175] that assigns a central role to beta-amyloid (Aβ), a small protein that is the main constituent of the plaques found in AD brains. Researchers have learned that Aβ is formed when APP is cut into small sections by enzymes called secretases. The factors that cause the disintegration of APP into Aβ fragments are a subject of active research. The Aβ plaques tend to clump together like a ball of spaghetti and form a mass outside brain cells. Advocates of the amyloid theory believe production and aggregation of Aβ to be the key event in the brain cell destruction process.

   The amyloid theory has led to several experimental treatment approaches. An early strategy for removing plaques involved immunizing AD patients with Aβ peptides to produce antibodies that can clear Aβ from the brain. An early vaccine[176] was successful in reducing plaques and improving mental functioning in mice. However, this therapy failed in human testing due to serious side effects. In a 2009 study, a different vaccine that had removed Aβ plaques in mice was given to 80 volunteer patients. The vaccine effectively reduced or completely eliminated the plaques in these persons. However, the researchers were disappointed to discover that removing the Aβ plaques had no measurable impact on the progressive destruction of brain cells and the course of the disease.[177] This finding suggests that Aβ plaques may be a result and not a cause of AD. A second amyloid-targeting strategy involves inhibition of the secretase enzymes that cut APP into fragments and produce Aβ. Several pharmaceutical companies are developing secretase inhibitors aimed at prevention of AD.

3. *The tau hypothesis:* The second most popular AD theory[178] assigns a primary role to tau, a protein that normally helps organize and stabilize a cell's internal skeleton. Tiny brain axons receive structural support from microtubules, tiny structures that resemble soda straws packed together. The microtubules also provide a conduit for vesicle and enzyme transport within the cell. Tau and other proteins assist in keeping the delicate tubules intact and in the proper place. However in AD patients, tau proteins become chemically modified and clump together, resulting in microtubule disintegration and disabling tangles. The net result is loss of nutrient transport and death of the brain cell. Figure 9-1 illustrates plaques and tangles observed in AD brain cells. Although no therapies targeting

Figure 9-1.

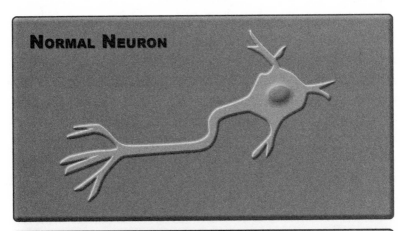

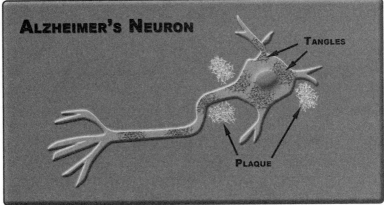

tau have reached clinical trials, many experts are convinced that understanding tau will reveal crucial clues about AD's devastating effects on nerve cells and lead to effective therapies.

4. ***Inflammation theory:*** In 2004, the Scripps Research Institute proposed a theory[179] that chronic inflammation is central to the development of AD. This theory was supported by mouse studies that found inflammation triggered a suspected AD mechanism and caused cognitive decline. The body's response to inflammation involves chemical changes, especially protein modifications. The Scripps theory suggests that amyloid proteins are modified during inflammation, causing them to misfold and accumulate into the characteristic plaques found in

AD brains. Scientists have launched several clinical trials to investigate whether anti-inflammatory drugs actually reduce AD risk. Other research groups are trying to identify molecular mechanisms that could explain protective effects of these drugs. Testing of primates has failed to confirm the findings of the Scripps mouse studies. Some experts believe anti-inflammatory therapies may have more application for AD prevention rather than addressing actual AD disease states.

5. *Oxidative stress theories:* There is considerable evidence[180-181] for the presence of excessive oxidative stress (free radicals) in AD brains. Oxidative free radicals perform several useful functions in the body, such as killing bacteria and burning glucose to produce energy. However, a chronic excess of free radicals can lead to death of brain cells. Sources of free radicals include physical injury, bacteria, viruses, inflammation, heavy metals, and nuclear radiation. The body has a supply of antioxidant molecules that have the job of keeping free radicals from reaching concentrations lethal to brain cells. A healthy brain requires (a) a competent blood-brain barrier to reduce influx of toxics, and (b) enough antioxidant protection within the brain to cope with the number of free radicals present. If the free radicals win the war, then neurodegeneration (death of brain cells) will occur.

Several antioxidant therapies have been the subject of formal studies, including vitamin E, vitamin E plus selenium, coenzyme Q10, glutathione, and lipoic acid. There is evidence[182] that some of these therapies increase the life span of AD patients but none has shown the ability to stop the advancing death of brain cells.

6. *Metal metabolism theories:* A number of research studies have implicated trace metal imbalances in the development of AD. Australian doctor Ashley Bush, MD, and colleagues[183] reported that copper overloads cause increased Aβ in the brain. Copper and iron are major sources of free radicals in the human brain, and elevated copper levels have been found in Aβ. Metallothionein and Cu/Zn SOD protect against copper free radicals, but both are depleted in AD brains. This theory suggests that excess copper prevents the natural removal of Aβ from AD brains. Interestingly, two 2009 studies[184-185] have reported a protective role for copper in AD. It's possible that either deficiency or excess of copper can be harmful to the brain and that homeostatic regulation of copper levels is essential.

Advanced Photon Source Measurements

In 2005, I organized a research study measuring metal concentrations in brain tissues from AD and age-matched control subjects. My collaborators were Barry Lai and Stefan Vogt of Argonne National Laboratory and Walter Lukiw of the Louisiana State University (LSU) Health Sciences Center. The tissues were 10-micron thick sections processed under highly stringent conditions at the LSU Neuroscience Center Brain Tissue Bank. The chemical assays were made at Argonne's Advanced Photon Source, using high-brilliance photon beams focused to 0.4 micron diameter. Samples were raster-scanned, yielding tens of thousands of individual measurements for zinc, copper, phosphorus, sulfur, chlorine, iron, aluminum, and calcium. Large calcium-rich circular areas were observed in the AD samples and very small calcium-rich zones in the controls. In both cases, the calcium concentrations were 15 times higher in the calcium-rich areas when compared with adjacent tissues.[186] Another interesting finding was the presence of very elevated Cu/Zn ratios in parts of the AD samples but not in the controls.

The Case for Metallothionein

Two separate autopsy studies[187-188] have reported severe deficiency of MT protein levels in deceased AD patients. MT proteins have several protective functions in the brain including the following:

- Preventing toxic metals from passing the blood-brain barrier
- Regulation of copper levels
- Powerful antioxidant action against free radicals

The protective properties of MT depend on ample amounts of glutathione and selenium, and I often refer to these antioxidants as the Three Musketeers. Gene expression of MT is zinc dependent, and most AD patients are depleted in zinc. MT proteins are far more powerful than selenium, coenzyme Q10, vitamins C and E, and other antioxidants that have been used in experimental AD therapies. In 2007, I received a US patent for an MT-Promotion formulation[147] for the treatment of autism, and a patent is pending for use of the same formulation for the treatment of AD. This formulation is comprised of 22 biochemical factors known to enhance the gene expression and functioning of MT. The treatment is a two-step process: normalization of plasma zinc levels followed by MT-Promotion therapy. A reliable caretaker is essential for treatment compliance since the AD patients may forget to take the capsules or take them repeatedly the same day. This treatment has been provided to more than 100 AD patients, resulting in many reports of improvement.

The first case involved an elderly Minnesota woman who had been diagnosed with AD and was a resident in a health care facility in the year 2000. She no longer remembered her grandchildren and was reported to have lost her sparkle and enthusiasm for life. After two months of MT-Promotion therapy, the family reported a partial return of memory and recognition of her grandchildren. They added that her irritability and malaise had disappeared and she wanted to go shopping. Her mental functioning remained fairly stable for the last seven years of her life.

Encouraged by this case history, we provided MT-Promotion therapy to increasing numbers of AD patients. In 2007, researcher Aditi Gulibani and I reviewed the progress of the first 60 AD patients who received MT-Promotion therapy. We learned that approximately 70% of the families reported a partial return of memory followed by stable mental functioning that continued for several years. In collaboration with Dr. John Crayton, CANTAB system testing was performed before and after treatment for dozens of patients, and in most cases, the data confirmed the reports of improved memory and stable cognitive function. Several of the improved patients were eventually told that they had been misdiagnosed, apparently since they hadn't deteriorated and died. Diagnosis of AD is preliminary prior to autopsy, so we cannot be certain that all of these patients actually had AD. It's also possible that some of the nonresponders had Lewy body disease or vascular dementia and not AD. In addition, the absence of a blinded control study means that the MT-Promotion approach must be regarded as unproven. Still, the positive reports from the first 100 persons treated with the MT-Promotion protocol suggests this approach is promising and worthy of additional study.

CHAPTER 10

THE CLINICAL PROCESS

Introduction

Advanced nutrient therapy involves a five-step process:

1. Medical history and review of symptoms
2. Lab testing of blood and urine
3. Diagnosis of chemical imbalance(s)
4. Treatment design
5. Aftercare

Each of these clinical steps is essential to treatment success. This therapy approach is complex and requires supervision by an experienced medical professional. Nutrient overloads or deficiencies can have a powerful effect on brain functioning and improper treatment can cause great harm. In other words: Don't try this at home! Find a doctor experienced in nutrient therapy!

Evolution of the Clinical System

In 1989, our clinical protocols were modeled after the system developed by Dr. Carl Pfeiffer at the Princeton Brain Bio Center in Skillman, New Jersey. Since that time, advances in brain science and biochemistry have produced numerous new treatment approaches. In most cases, we performed outcome studies to measure treatment effectiveness prior to incorporation into our clinical protocols. This activity yielded several disappointments as well as many successes. For example, we confidently began supplementing low-histamine patients with histidine, the amino acid that converts to histamine in the body. Unfortunately, this often produced dramatic worsening, and the procedure was discontinued after discovering that histidine supplements caused severe zinc deficiency in these patients.

In another misadventure, we began treating manganese-deficient Tourette syndrome patients with manganese supplements. This resulted in lower dopamine activity and made symptoms worse. An example of a successful trial involved use of SAMe for undermethylated depressed patients in 1991. It didn't take long to learn that SAMe produced more rapid improvements than any previous methylation approach. Brain biochemistry is very complex, and each new therapy or clinical procedure must be put to the test. This evaluation approach has brought great improvements in reported outcomes since 1990, and future advances will be achieved as additional mysteries of brain biochemistry are resolved.

Medical History and Review of Symptoms

Successful nutrient therapy requires in-depth knowledge of the patient, and an extensive medical history is essential. Lab chemistries provide only 50% of the information needed for accurate diagnosis. Each biochemical imbalance is associated with a distinctive collection of physical characteristics and behavioral traits, and it is often possible to predict the lab findings before testing. The ideal situation occurs when symptoms and traits dovetail with the blood and urine chemistries. Table 10-1 presents a partial list of medical history factors that can assist in diagnosis.

Some patients become discouraged if they have a close relative with the same

---

Table 10-1.
Medical History Factors

Problems during pregnancy	Problems during birth
Early health issues	Food sensitivities
Developmental milestones	Growth history
Seasonal allergies	Chemical sensitivities
Illnesses	Injuries
Academic strengths and weaknesses	Academic level
Family unit	Occupation
Medical diagnoses and treatments	Response to medications
Immune function	Behavior control
OCD tendencies	Sleep issues
Substance abuse issues	Pain threshold
Family history of illnesses	Socialization issues
Competitiveness	Diet

mental disorder. They assume their condition may be inevitable and untreatable since it appears genetic in nature. Over the years, I've learned the exact opposite is true: the best treatment candidates are those with a family history of the same disorder. An inherited mental illness usually involves abnormal brain chemistry, and chemistry can be adjusted. The prospects are poorer for patients who experienced a difficult birth or a severe head injury.

In our early clinical experience, we were surprised to learn that more than 30% of violent children receiving our services had been adopted, and this population generally had better outcomes than other children with behavioral disorders. We believe a high percentage of the adoptees inherited abnormal brain chemistry from dysfunctional birth parents but were adopted by caring and capable persons who sought solutions when problems developed. Typically, the adoptees had a striking combination of terrible chemistry and an excellent family environment. Most of these families reported a complete elimination of violent episodes following nutrient therapy.

Telltale Clues of a Chemical Imbalance

The primary nutrient imbalances that impact mental health are usually accompanied by a distinctive set of symptoms and traits. This information can be valuable in forming a correct diagnosis, especially when chemistry findings are inconclusive. General syndromes associated with these imbalances are summarized below. The presence of more than 30% of these symptoms and traits is considered a positive indication of the imbalance.

Zinc deficiency: Poor growth through puberty with significant growth after age 16, white spots on fingernails, frequent infections, tendency for sunburn, preference for spicy foods, irritability, poor stress control, anger, poor wound healing, poor muscle development, premature graying of hair, abnormal or absent menstrual periods, stretch marks on skin.

Copper overload: Hyperactivity, academic underachievement, skin sensitivity to metals and rough fabrics, estrogen intolerance, emotional meltdowns, ringing in ears, sensitivity to food dyes, high anxiety, sleep problems, adverse reaction to nutritional supplements containing copper, abnormal menstrual periods.

Undermethylation: Obsessive-compulsive tendencies, seasonal allergies, strong-willed, competitive in games and sports, ritualistic behaviors, high libido, poor pain tolerance, addictive tendencies, sparse arm/leg/chest hair, history of perfectionism, chronic depression, high fluidity (tears, saliva), phobias.

Overmethylation: High anxiety; dry eyes and mouth; hirsutism; noncompetitive; low libido; talkative; low motivation in early school years; obsessions without compulsive actions; sleep disorder; food and chemical sensitivities; estrogen intolerance; absence of seasonal allergies; postpartum depression; antihistamine intolerance; adverse reaction to SSRI antidepressants, methionine, and SAMe.

Pyrrole disorder: Poor stress control, poor short-term memory, reading disorder, sensitivity to noise and bright lights, little or no dream recall, spleen area pain, poor growth, many fears, dry skin, underachievement, tendency to skip breakfast, frequent infections, extreme mood swings, severe inner tension, abnormal fat distribution, affinity for spicy or salty foods, high anxiety, delayed puberty, abnormal EEG.

Toxic metal overload: Abdominal discomfort, poor appetite, increased irritability and temper, decline in academics, metallic taste in mouth, bad breath, change in personality.

Although the above information is helpful in forming a diagnosis, it should be considered inconclusive in the absence of blood and urine testing. The combination of a good medical history and reliable lab testing is essential to accurate diagnosis.

Laboratory Testing

There are a multitude of lab assays that can provide valid evidence of disordered brain chemistry. However, if patients had every available test, they wouldn't have a drop of blood left and probably no money either. Clearly, it is necessary to make priorities in lab testing. My approach has been to establish a basic test portfolio that enables accurate diagnosis for most patients, with additional assays performed in complex cases. There are several labs in the USA and elsewhere that capably perform these tests. If possible, samples should be submitted to labs with CLIA certification to maximize the chances of high proficiency. Some of useful laboratory tests are described below:

+ *Whole blood histamine:* This is a useful test for evaluating methylation status. Histamine and methyl groups are present in measurable levels throughout the body, and an inverse relationship exists between them. Histamine is metabolized (destroyed) by methylation, and this is a primary mechanism for regulating histamine concentrations. Elevated blood histamine indicates undermethylation, and low histamine is evidence of overmethylation. Antihistamine treatments can artificially lower blood histamine and should be avoided for several days prior to sampling. Laboratory assays for SAMe/SAH ratio are more decisive, but they are not widely available in commercial laboratories.

+ *Plasma zinc:* There are about 10 different approaches for measuring zinc status, and plasma testing has consistently been regarded by zinc experts as the best way to obtain reliable and meaningful results. The zinc concentration in blood serum is nearly identical, but this approach involves a greater likelihood of contamination during sampling. Some doctors prefer to assay packed cells, which gives an indication of the zinc level within blood cells rather than in blood fluids. Testing of both plasma and blood cells provides additional information that is sometimes useful in diagnosis.

+ *Serum copper:* This is a routine and highly reliable assay that is available in many parts of the world. Copper has special significance in mental health due to its role in metabolism of dopamine and synthesis of norepinephrine (see Chapter 3). Elevated serum copper can alter the synaptic activity of these important neurotransmitters.

+ *Urine pyrroles:* This chemical assay is available in laboratories in the USA, Europe, and Australia and is gaining in popularity. This test serves two purposes:

  ▪ Identification of pyrrole disorder, a medical condition associated with extreme deficiencies of B-6 and zinc
  ▪ Assessment of oxidative stress in an individual

Pyrrole disorder typically involves high anxiety, poor behavioral control, a reading disorder, impaired immune function, and other troubling symptoms. Severe pyrrole levels have been observed in persons diagnosed with violent behaviors, depression, schizophrenia, and other serious mental disorders. Elevated pyrroles can also result from excessive oxidative stress levels in persons who do not have the classic symptoms and traits of pyrrole disorder.

- *Serum ceruloplasmin:* In healthy individuals, about 80 to 95% of serum copper is bound to ceruloplasmin, with the remaining 5-20% present as loosely bound atoms or unbound free radicals. Patients with more than 25% of their copper not bound to ceruloplasmin have a metal metabolism disorder involving elevated oxidative stress. This condition is common in autism, postpartum depression, ADHD, and certain forms of psychosis.

- *Thyroid panel:* A surprisingly high number of patients with chemical imbalances also exhibit hypothyroidism. Normalizing thyroid levels is essential to treatment success for these persons. In rare cases, hypothyroidism alone can cause clinical depression or psychosis.

- *Liver enzymes:* The presence of elevated liver enzymes suggests this organ is under significant stress, and nutrient therapy should be modified to avoid aggravating the condition. Liver enzyme elevations are a common side effect of psychiatric medications. In any case, high dosages of niacinamide and fat-soluble vitamins such as A, D, and E should be avoided for these patients.

Think Neurotransmitters!

Most mental illnesses involve abnormal synaptic activity of one or more brain neurotransmitters, and treatment design should reflect this reality. For example, undermethylated patients generally have depressed serotonin activity, and treatment should provide nutrients that elevate serotonin activity and avoid those that depress it. Table 10-2 shows the impact of specific nutrients for some of the primary neurotransmitters.

Aftercare

Open communication with families is a high priority, especially during the first few months of treatment. Common issues include compliance difficulties, temporary adverse side effects, psychiatric medications, and a more healthful, therapeutic diet. Many of these problems can be resolved without involving a physician. My favorite approach is for each patient to have a primary care nurse who can provide practical

---

Table 10-2.
Neurotransmitter-Nutrient Relationships

	Increased Activity	Decreased Activity
Serotonin	Methionine, SAMe, 5-HTP, tryptophan, inositol, Ca, Mg, vitamins B-2, B-6, D	Folic acid, DMAE, choline, vitamin B-5, niacinamide, CoA
Dopamine	Tyrosine, phenylalanine, vitamins B-1, B-6, SAMe, methionine	Folic acid, vitamins B-5, C, choline, DMAE, niacinamide, Mn, GABA, CoA
Norepinephrine	Tyrosine, phenylalanine, copper, vitamins B-6, C	GABA, folic acid, DMAE, niacinamide, Mg, CoA, zinc, vitamin B-5, choline
NMDA	Glutamine, glutathione, glycine, D-Cycloserine, sarcosine, D-Serine, Se	Low glycine level, low glutathione level, high oxidative stress
GABA	Pyridoxyl-5-Phosphate, zinc	Aspartic acid

suggestions to cope with such difficulties. If a complex medical issue is involved, the nurse can bring the doctor into the discussion. Another requirement for effective aftercare is regular checkups with the doctor. Patients with ADHD, BD, or mental illness should be retested after three to six months to enable fine-tuning of dosages, with follow-up about once annually thereafter. In my experience, children with autism should be evaluated every six months until age six.

Treatment Compliance

Poor compliance is the most frequent cause of treatment failure. To facilitate compliance, doctors should make treatments as simple as possible by minimizing the number of capsules needed and the frequency of dosing. Nutrient therapy requires the patient to swallow capsules, tablets, or powders containing the prescribed nutrients. Most children under the age of 6 have difficulty with capsules or tablets, but they can ingest powders stirred into juice or other acceptable fluids. Most children are able to swallow capsules and tablets after age six, but there are many exceptions. A compounding pharmacy can usually reduce the number of capsules by a factor of two to three, which can make all the difference for patients with compliance issues. Several key nutrients have a very unpleasant taste, and many pharmacies offer innocuous additives (such as vanillin) that can mask the unpleasant taste.

Typically, patients are asked to take some nutrients with breakfast and others with the evening meal. Vitamin B-6 is a component of most treatments and can make sleep difficult if taken late in the day. For patients who are intolerant of morning nutrients, we recommend vitamin B-6 be taken prior to 3:30 pm. About 25% of patients taking zinc in the morning (or without food) report nausea or stomach pain. For this reason, zinc is usually given with the evening meal. Absorption efficiency drops somewhat for certain nutrients if taken at mealtime. The doctor can adjust for this effect by prescribing small increases in dosage.

Many persons with pyrrole disorder report little or no appetite in the morning and avoid breakfast entirely. For these patients, we recommend the morning nutrients be taken with the first substantial meal.

More than 50% of patients exhibit a dominant chemical imbalance that is the cause of their illness. In these cases, treatment should concentrate on that imbalance and avoid adjustments of other biochemical factors or special diets until significant progress is achieved. An exception is made for patients with autism who require multiple therapies and are sensitive to dietary casein and gluten.

Some first-time patients report awful diets that require major improvements. I recall a bipolar patient who reported his diet in the past 30 days consisted of tortilla chips and cola from vending machines. In my experience, better outcomes are achieved if the primary imbalance is corrected before dietary intervention begins. Many patients are unable to make a major change in lifestyle before the major imbalance is corrected. A nutritional practitioner needs to grit his/her teeth and avoid major dietary changes until treatment progress is achieved. In an exception, ADHD children should limit sweets and restrict food dyes at the outset. Another exception involves children diagnosed with ASD who need special diets from the initial stages of treatment.

Oppositional and Defiant Patients

Many children and teenagers diagnosed with ADHD or BD have little or no interest in medical interventions and plan to sabotage treatment. An effective approach is to spend considerable time alone with them to identify a treatment benefit they might want. If a child is below average in height, the conversation might center on the fact that zinc deficiency can stunt growth. Children involved in sports might become motivated upon learning that world-class athletes have reported benefits from our nutrient therapy. We rejoice if an oppositional teenage girl presents with acne since that attitude may change after discovering that treatment clears the complexion. Violent children sometimes cooperate when told our objective is to put them in complete control of their actions. Some oppositional-defiant patients will agree to a treatment trial of a few months if, after this time, THEY are allowed to decide if life is better and whether to continue. In nearly every case, oppositional-defiant children will find a way to sabotage compliance unless they believe they can benefit in some way.

Direct Interaction with Psychotic Patients

Many practitioners prefer to obtain medical history information from family members in the absence of the patient, who may be angry and disruptive. However, after collecting medical histories for 2,000 schizophrenics, I've learned the great value in meeting directly with the patient and getting as much information from him/her as possible. Many patients are paranoid and imagine that private discussions with parents involve plans for institutionalization or lobotomy. It's best to invite full participation by the patient, which builds teamwork, confidence, and improves the likelihood of treatment compliance.

Patients Taking Concerta, Adderal, or Ritalin

Many ADHD and BD patients report ongoing treatment with an amphetamine medication during the initial evaluation. Outcome studies have shown best results are attained if the medication is continued during the first three to six months of nutrient therapy. After that time, we suggest the family ask the psychiatrist to gradually reduce doses until an optimum condition is reached. About 80% of these families report medication can be reduced to zero without symptoms returning. The remaining 20% of families report that some benefits are lost when the amphetamine is eliminated. In this event, the drug dosage has usually been reduced (with lessened side effects), and we recommend continuation of both therapies.

Substance Abuse

After many failed attempts, I learned that patients currently abusing cocaine, heroin, and other illegal drugs have a zero treatment success rate from nutrient therapy. However, significant progress is possible if the patient has abstained from the drug for at least six weeks. Marijuana is an exception, with many cases of treatment success even if this drug abuse is continued. Also, new research[189] strongly indicates that

N-acetylcysteine (NAC) reduces cocaine cravings and can assist in treatment of addicted patients.

Similarly, alcoholic patients who continue drinking during nutrient therapy rarely improve. Nearly all patients underestimate their alcohol intake, and a general rule is to multiply their reported intake by a factor of three. Complete abstinence for at least six weeks should precede nutrient therapy. Alcohol abuse is known to diminish glutamate activity at NMDA receptors,[190-191] and nutrients that enhance NMDA function are an important part of therapy. These include vitamin B-6, zinc, sarcosine, D-serine, and D-cycloserine.

Nutrient Therapy Side Effects

If the biochemical diagnosis is incorrect, an improper nutrient therapy can cause great harm. In some cases, certain sensitive patients can experience significant adverse reactions even if the diagnosis is correct. Adverse reactions may be divided into three types: (a) side effects resulting from rapid biochemical transitions during early treatment, (b) symptoms associated with extreme nutrient sensitivities, and (c) adverse reactions associated with incorrect diagnosis or excessive nutrient dosages.

a. *Transitional side effects:* Many patients exhibit an overload of copper or a toxic metal prior to treatment. These excess materials depart the body via the bloodstream during early nutrient therapy. If the exit from the body is too rapid, blood levels can escalate and cause unpleasant side effects. Other side effects can occur if excess histamine is released too rapidly from tissues. In all cases of transitional side effects, the solution is to take one's foot off the accelerator and temporarily reduce treatment dosages.

b. *Nutrient sensitivities:* There is great individuality with respect to nutrient sensitivities, and doctors should be alert for these rare side effects. Some patients are very sensitive to nutrients that are in deficiency. For example, many children with autism are deficient in cysteine, glutathione, and other sulfur-containing nutrients, but they exhibit extreme negative reactions during modest dosages. Human biochemistry is complex, and there are a multitude of genetic variations between different persons. Occasional unexpected results of nutrient therapy are inevitable.

c. *Incorrect therapy:* Nutrient therapy should be supervised by a medical professional with experience in this medical approach. An example of improper treatment is excessive zinc dosage that can produce anemia due to reduction in iron stores. Manganese incorrectly given to an undermethylated patient can produce Parkinsonian-like symptoms. Patients with vitamin B-6 sufficiency can develop temporary skin neuropathy and wild troubling dreams after doses of vitamin B-6. Undermethylated patients can develop worsened depression and psychotic symptoms if mistakingly given folic acid. Overmethylated patients may develop worsened anxiety and depression if given methionine or SAMe methylating agents. Treatment with copper can increase the risk of hormonal cancers in high-copper females. Individualized nutrient therapy should never be attempted by inexperienced lay persons.

Dosage-Weight Relationship

The optimal nutrient dose for a small child would be insufficient for a large adult sharing the identical chemical imbalance. In addition to weight, a person's area/ volume ratio affects nutritional equivalency. Nutritional scientists use a metabolic weight factor (MWF) that enables more precise dosing for persons of different body weight. MWF is approximately equal to the weight ratio taken to the 0.75 power. In essence, smaller persons require a higher mg/kg dose than larger persons. For example a 26-pound child needs about 25% of the dose for a 160-pound adult for nutritional equivalency, although the child's weight is only 16% of 160 lbs. Similarly, a 320-pound adult requires less than half the dosage required for a 160-pound person. This system is useful in selecting initial treatment dosages. Follow-up lab testing after a few months of therapy can determine the degree of chemical imbalance and enable fine-tuning of dosages.

Dosage for Malabsorbers

About 10% of patients are malabsorbers who process foods and nutritional supplements with low efficiency. These patients need higher nutrient doses to normalize body chemistry. My general rule is to increase dosages by 10%, 20%, or 30% for persons with mild, moderate, or severe malabsorption, respectively.

Stress Dosing

Patients with a history of zinc deficiency have a tendency to relapse during a prolonged, stressful period. Over the years we have learned that temporary increases of zinc can be very useful in maintaining treatment effectiveness. I recall a patient who increased her zinc dosage before visits from her mother-in-law.

Nutrient Therapy Response Times

The response to nutrient therapy is relatively slow when compared with that of psychiatric medications. In addition, response times vary greatly for different chemical imbalances. Typical treatment response times (assuming good compliance) are shown below for some of the major biochemical imbalances.

- *Pyrrole disorder:* Nice improvement in behavior control and calming can be seen during week one, with full effectiveness after one month.

- *Zinc deficiency:* Little improvement is seen during the first two weeks, with gradual improvement thereafter and full effectiveness after 60 days.

- *Copper overload:* There are many reports of mild worsening during the first 10 days, followed by clear improvement during weeks three and four and full effectiveness after three to four months (except in the case of type A blood, which may require 6-12 months for full effectiveness).

- *Overmethylation:* There is increased anxiety during the first two to three weeks, followed by sharp improvement during weeks four to eight and full effectiveness after three to four months.

- *Undermethylation:* Little/no improvement is seen during the first three to four weeks, followed by steady improvement during months two to six.

- *Toxic metal overload:* There is mild worsening during the first 10 days, followed by steady improvement for four to six months. Removal of lead is especially slow (half-life of long-term lead in the body is 22 years). Other metal toxins can be removed relatively quickly.

Factors that often retard progress are malabsorption, type A blood, and hypoglycemia. Patients who have all three factors require great patience since initial progress can be delayed by several months. In addition, treatment response usually is very protracted for treatment of undermethylated schizophrenia and bipolar patients. For these persons, improvement usually begins after 3 to 6 weeks, with 12 months often needed for the full effect.

Nonresponders

As with all medical therapies, there are some patients who fail to improve after nutrient therapy. While working with 30,000 patients, I encountered numerous cases in which little or no improvement was reported despite promising biochemistry. Careful analysis of nonresponders has identified the 10 most frequent reasons for treatment failure:

1. *Noncompliance:* More than 50% of all treatment failures resulted from poor treatment compliance. About 10% of oppositional children and teens refused to comply, and some never took a single capsule. We learned that many children can be adept at sleight of hand and avoid compliance without the parents' knowledge. We received many reports of flower pots filled with soggy capsules. I believe the honor system is unwise for ADHD or children with behavioral disorders.

2. *Growth spurt:* Some zinc-deficient patients experience rapid growth during the first few months of treatment and fail to improve until the growth spurt has ended. We use and lose zinc when cells divide, and standard zinc doses are insufficient if rapid growth occurs.

3. *Physical injury:* Successfully treated patients may experience a temporary relapse after a broken leg or similar injury. If an injury occurs during early treatment, symptoms may worsen for weeks before progress is noted.

4. *Illness:* Infections and other illnesses can result in biochemical changes that may delay response to treatment.

5. *Emotional stress:* Several chemical imbalances are heightened during traumatic experiences. I recall an ADHD child who failed to respond after months of good compliance. His mother discovered he was being terrorized daily by a school bully, and his academics improved nicely after the situation was resolved.

6. *Type A blood:* Outcome studies indicate that persons with type A blood respond very slowly to nutrient therapy. The combination of a metal metabolism disorder and type A blood can require great patience on the part of the family.

7. *Malabsorption:* Persons who process foods inefficiently usually have a slowed response to nutrient therapy.

8. *Anoxia during birth:* Patients with a history of oxygen deprivation during birth were found to have an increased probability of treatment failure.

9. *Head injuries:* Persons with a history of serious head injury have an increased incidence of treatment failure.

10. *Substance abuse:* Many nonresponding patients eventually were discovered to have been secretly abusing alcohol or illegal drugs during treatment. Serious substance abuse usually nullifies the benefits of nutrient therapy.

For every person who does not respond to nutrient therapy, there are many more who report major improvements and achieve a higher quality of life. The treatment approaches described in this book are relatively safe and free of adverse side effects. As biochemical science progresses, great improvements in treatment effectiveness will be achieved with this modality. I believe we are approaching a new enlightened era in mental health in which therapies will be aimed at normalizing brain function rather than introducing foreign molecules into the brain. Every human being deserves the opportunity to achieve the highest attainable degree of health, safety, function, and happiness, and this approach is the best way to reach this goal. Progress in epigenetics will enable future cures for many mental and developmental disorders, and epigenetics research must become a high national priority.

REFERENCES

1. Larson RM. (2004). *Science in the Ancient World: An Encyclopedia.* ABC-CLIO: Santa Barbara, CA; 29-30.

2. Debus AG. (1970). Johann Hoachim Becher. In: Gillispie CC, ed. *Dictionary of Scientific Biography.* Vol. 1. Charles Scribner's Sons: New York.

3. Conant JB, ed. (1950). *The Overthrow of Phlogiston Theory: The Chemical Revolution of 1775-1789.* Harvard University Press: Cambridge, MA; 14.

4. Thompson JJ. (1904). On the structure of the atom: an investigation of the stability and periods of oscillation of a number of corpuscles arranged at equal intervals around the circumference of a circle; with application of the results to the theory of atomic structure. *Philos Magazine,* Series 6. 7(39):237-265.

5. Winkler KP, ed. (1996). *John Locke, An Essay Concerning Human Understanding.* Hackett Publishing Company: Indianapolis, IN; 33-36.

6. Aristotle (350 BC). *On the soul (de anima).* In: *Aristotle.* Vol. 8 (1936). Hett, WS, trans. Loeb Classical Library, William Heinemann: London; 1-203.

7. Freud S. (1940). An outline of psycho-analysis (the standard edition). In: Strachey J, ed. *Complete Psychological Works of Sigmund Freud.* W W Norton: New York.

8. Adler A. (1956). In: Ansbacher, HL and Ansbacher RR, eds. *The Individual Psychology of Alfred Adler.* Harper Torchbooks: New York.

9. Kendler KS. (1983). Overview: a current perspective on twin studies of schizophrenia. *Am J Psychiatry.* 140:1413-1425.

10. Bertelsen A, Harvald B, Hauge M. (1977). A Danish twin study of manic-depressive disorders. *Br J Psychiatry.* 130:330-351.

11. Wender PH, Kety SS, Rosenthal D, Schulsinger F, Ortmann J, Lunde I. (1986). Psychiatric disorders in the biological and adoptive families of adopted individuals with affective disorders. *Arch Gen Psychiatry.* 43:923-929.

12. Snyder SH. (1986). *Drugs and the Brain.* Scientific American Books/WH Freeman: New York.

13. Purves D, Augustine GJ, Fitzpatrick D, et al. (2004). *Neuroscience.* 4th ed. Sinauer Associates, Inc.: Sunderland, MA.

14. Restak RM. (1984). *The Brain.* Bantam Books: New York.

15. Qian Y, Melikian HE, Rye DB, Levey AI, Blakely RD. (1995). Identification and characterization of antidepressant-sensitive serotonin transporter proteins using site-specific antibodies. *J Neurosci.* 15:1261-1274.

16. Torres GE, Gainetdinov RR, Caron MG. (2003). Plasma membrane monoamine transporters: structure, regulation and function. *Nat Rev Neurosci.* 4(1):13-25.

17. Wade NJ, Brozek J. (2001). *Purkinje's Vision–The Dawning of Neuroscience.* Lawrence Erlbaum Assoc.: London.

18. Golgi C. (1906). In: *Nobel Lectures, Physiology or Medicine 1901-1921.* (1967). Elsevier Publishing Company: Amsterdam.

19. Cajal R. (1906). In: *Nobel Lectures, Physiology or Medicine 1901-1921.* (1967). Elsevier Publishing Company: Amsterdam.

20. Sherrington CS. (1920). *The Integrative Action of the Nervous System.* New Haven Yale Press: New Haven, CT.

21. Raju TN. (1999). The Nobel chronicles. 1936: Henry Hallett Dale (1875-1968) and Otto Loewi (1873-1961). *Lancet.* 353(9150): 416.

22. Fields DR (2009). *The Other Brain.* Simon & Schuster: New York.

23. Rizzoli SO, Betz WJ (2005). Synaptic vesicle pools. *Nat Rev Neurosci.* 6(1):57-69.

24. Weihe E, Eiden LE. (2000). Chemical neuroanatomy of the vesicular amine transporters. *FASEB J.* 14(15):2435-2449.

25. Hoffer A. (2005). *Adventures in Psychiatry. The Scientific Memoirs of Dr. Abram Hoffer.* KOS Publishing: Toronto.

26. Wittenborn JR, Weber ESP, Brown M. (1973). Niacin in the long-term treatment of schizophrenia. *Arch Gen Psychiatry.* 28:308-315.

27. McGinnis W, Audhya T, Walsh WJ, et al. (2008). Discerning the mauve factor, part 1. *Altern Ther Health Med.* 14(2):40-50.

28. Pfeiffer CC. (1976). *Mental and Elemental Nutrients: A Physician's Guide to Nutrition and Health Care.* Keats Publishing: New Canaan, CT.

29. Pfeiffer CC, Mailloux BS, Forsythe BA. (1970). *The Schizophrenias: Ours to conquer.* Bio-Communications Press: Wichita, KS.

30. Walsh WJ, Glab LB, Haakenson ML. (2004). Reduced violent behavior following biochemical therapy. *Physiol Behav.* 82:835-839.

31. Owen CA. (1982). *Biochemical aspects of copper, occurrence, assay, and interrelationships.* Noyes Publications: Park Ridge, NJ.

32. Linder MC. (1991). *Biochemistry of Copper.* Plenum Press: New York.

33. Morgan RF, O'Dell BL. (1977). Effect of copper deficiency on the concentrations of catecholamines and related enzyme activities in the rat brain. *J Neurochem.* 28:207-213.

34. Prohaska JR, Snith TL. (1982). Effect of dietary or genetic copper deficiency on brain catecholamines, trace metals, and enzymes in the rat brain. *J Nutr.* 112:1706-1717.

35. Combs GF. (2008). *The Vitamins: Fundamental Aspects in Nutrition and Health.* Elsevier: San Diego, CA.

36. Food and Nutrition Board, Institute of Medicine. (2001). *Dietary Reference Intakes: Vitamins.* The National Academies Press: Washington, DC.

37. Berger M, Gray JA, Roth BL. (2009). The expanded biology of serotonin. *Ann Rev Med.* 60:355-366.

38. Elsworth JD, Roth RH. (1997). Dopamine synthesis, uptake, metabolism, and receptors: relevance to gene therapy of Parkinson's disease. *Exp Neurol.* 144(1): 4-9.

39. Tapia R. (1975). Biochemical pharmacology of GABA in CNS. In: Iversen LL, Iversen SD, Snyder SH, eds. *Handbook of Psychopharmacology.* Vol 4. Plenum Press: New York; 1-58.

40. Sauberlich HE. (1999). *Laboratory Tests for the Assessment of Nutritional Status.* CRC Press: New York.

41. Prasad AS. (1993). *Biochemistry of Zinc.* Plenum Press: New York.

42. Walsh WJ, Rehman F. (1997). Methylation syndromes in mental illness. *Abstracts: Society for Neuroscience 27th Annual Meeting* (pt 2). New Orleans, LA, October 25-29.

43. Feighner JP. (1999). Mechanism of action of antidepressant medications. *J Clin Psychiatry.* 60(suppl 4):4-11.

44. Edelman E. (2009). *Natural Healing for Bipolar Disorder.* Borage Books: Eugene, OR.

45. Murray RK, Granner DK, Mayes PA, Rodwell VW. (1993). *Harper's Biochemistry.* 23rd ed. Appleton & Lange: Norwalk, CT; 49-59.

46. Berger SL, Kouzarides T, Schickhatter R, Shilatifard A. (2009). *An operational definition of epigenetics. Genes Dev.* 23(7):781-783.

47. Bird A. (2007). Perceptions of epigenetics. *Nature.* 447(7143):396-398.

48. Tsankova N, Renthal W, Kumar A, Nestler EJ. (2007). Epigenetic regulation in psychiatric disorders. *Nat Rev Neurosci.* 8(5):355-367.

49. Ng HH, Gurdon JB. (2008). Epigenetic inheritance of cell differentiation status. *Cell Cycle.* 7(9):1173-1177.

50. Luger K, Mader AW, Richmond RK, Sargent DF, Richmond TJ. (1997). Crystal structure of the nucleosome core particle at 2.8 A resolution. *Nature.* 389(6648):251-260.

51. Roth TL, Sodhi M, Kleinmer JE. (2009). Epigenetic mechanisms in schizophrenia. *Biochem Biophy Acta.* 1790(9):869-877.

52. Flight M. (2007). Epigenetics: methylation and schizophrenia. *Nat Rev Neurosci.* 8:910-994.

53. Suzuki MM, Bird AP. (2008). DNA methylation landscapes: provocative insights from epigenomics. *Nat Rev. Genet.* 9(6):465-476.

54. Kouzarides T. (2007). Chromatin modifications and their function. *Cell.* 128(4):693-705.

55. Miranda TB, Jones PA. (2007). DNA methylation: The nuts and bolts of repression. *J Cell Physiol.* 213(2):384-390.

56. Latchman DS. (1997). Transcription factors: an overview. *Int J Biochem. Cell Biol.* 29(12):1305-1312.

57. Nelson DL, Cox MM. (2000). *Lehninger Principles of Biochemistry.* 3rd ed. Worth Publishing: New York.

58. Avalos JL, Bever KM, Wolberger C. (2005). Mechanism of sirtuin inhibition by nicotinamide: altering the NAD+ cosubstrate specificity of a Sir2 enzyme. *Mol Cell.* 17(6):855-868.

59. Luka Z, Moss F, Loukachevitch LV, Bornhop DJ, Wagner C. (2011). Histone demethylase LSD1 is a folate-binding protein. *Biochemistry.* 50(21):4750-4756.

60. Jenuwein T, Allis CD. (2001). Translating the histone code. *Science.* 293(5532):1074-1080.

61. Preskorn SH, Ross R, Stanga CY. (2004). Selective serotonin reuptake inhibitors. In: *Antidepressants: Past, Present and Future.* Springer: Berlin; 241-262.

62. Sharma RP. (2005). Schizophrenia, epigenetics and ligand-activated nuclear reactions: a framework for chromatin therapeutics. *Schizophr Res.* 72(2-3):77-90.

63. Petronis A. (2004). The origin of schizophrenia: genetic thesis, epigenetic antithesis, and resolving synthesis. *Biol Psychiatry.* 55:965-970.

64. Bilstufi G, VanDette E, Matsui S, Smiraglia DJ. (2010). Mild folate deficiency induces genetic and epigenetic instability and phenotype changes in prostate cancer cells. *BMC Biol.* 8:6.

65. Maulik N, Maulik G, eds. (2011). *Nutrition, Epigenetic Mechanisms, and Human Disease.* CRC Press: Boca Raton, FL.

66. Pogribny IP, Tryndyak VP, Muskhelishvili L, Rusyn I, Ross SA. (2007). Methyl deficiency, alterations in global histone modifications, and carcinogenesis. *J Nutr.* 137:216S-222S.

67. Litt MD, Simpson M, Recillas-Targa F, Prioleau MN, Felsenfeld G. (2001). Transitions in histone acetylation reveal boundaries of three separately regulated neighboring loci. *EMBO J.* 20(9):2224-2235.

68. Bredy TW, Sun Ye, Kobor MS. (2010). How the epigenome contributes to the development of psychiatric disorders. *Dev Psychobiol.* 52(4):331-342.

69. James SJ, Melnyk SB, Jernigan S, Janak L, Cutler P, Neubrander JM. (2004). Metabolic biomarkers of increased oxidative stress and impaired methylation capacity in children with autism. *Amer J Clin Nutr.* 80:1611-1117.

70. Deth RC. (2003). *Molecular Origins of Attention: The Dopamine-Folate Connection.* Kluwer Academic Publishers: Norwell, MA.

71. Walsh WJ. (2010). Oxidative stress, undermethylation, and epigenetics—The Bermuda triangle of autism. *The Autism File.* 35:30-35.

72. Walsh WJ. (July 23, 2010). Nutrient therapy for mental illness. *Irish Medical Times.* Available at www.imt.ie/opinion/guests/2010/07/nutrient-therapy-for-mental-illness. html.

73. American Psychiatric Association. (2000). *Diagnostic and statistical manual of mental disorders, Fourth Edition (Text Revision).* American Psychiatric Press: Washington, DC.

74. Jablonka E, Gal R. (2009). Transgenerational Epigenetic Inheritance: Prevalence, Mechanisms, and Implications for the Study of Heredity and Evolution. *Q Rev Biol.* 84(2):131-176.

75. Evans K, McGrath J, Milns R. (2003). Searching for schizophrenia in ancient Greek and Roman literature: a systematic review. *Acta Psychiatrica Scandinavica.* 107(5):323-330.

76. Alexander FG, Selesnick ST. (1966). *The History of Psychiatry. An Evaluation of Psychiatric Thought and Practice from Prehistoric Times to the Present.* Harper and Row: New York.

77. Kruger S, Braunig P. (2000). Ewald Hecker, 1843-1900. *Am J Psychiatry.* 157:1220.

78. Meyer A. (1910). The nature and conception of dementia praecox. *J Abnorm Psychol.* 5(5):247-285.

79. Kraepelin E. (1907). *Text book of psychiatry.* 7th ed. Diefendorf AR, trans. Macmillan: London.

80. Kuhn R. (2004). Eugen Bleuler's concepts of psychopathology. *Hist Psychiatry.* 15(3):361-366.

81. Freud S, trans, Brill AA. (1938). *The Basic Writings by Sigmund Freud.* Random House: New York.

82. Adler A, trans, Brett C. (1992). *Understanding Human Nature.* Oneworld Publications Ltd.: London.

83. Jung CJ, trans, Adler G, Hull RFC. (1970). *The Collected Works of C. J. Jung.* Vol 1. Princeton University Press: Princeton, NJ.

84. Schildkraut JJ. (1965). The catecholamine hypothesis of affective disorders: a review of supporting evidence. *Amer J Psychiatry.* 122:609-622.

85. Slater E, Cowle V. (1971). *The Genetics of Mental Disorders.* Oxford University Press: London.

86. Mathews M, Muzina DJ. (2007). Atypical antipsychotics: new drugs, new challenges. *Cleve Clin J Med.* 74(8):597-606.

87. Lieberman JA, Stroup TS, McEvoy JP, et al. (2005). Effectiveness of antipsychotic drugs in patients with chronic schizophrenia. *NEJM.* 353(12):1209-1223.

88. Ho BC, Andersen NC, Ziebell S, Pierson R, Magnotta V. (2011). Long-term antipsychotic treatment and brain volumes: a longitudinal study of first-episode schizophrenia. *Arch Gen Psych.* 68:2.

89. Carlsson A. (2003). Half-century of neurotransmitter research: impact on neurology and psychiatry. In: Jörnvall H, ed. *Nobel Lectures in Physiology or Medicine 1996-2000.* World Scientific Publishing Co.: Singapore.

90. Carlsson A. (1987). The dopamine hypothesis of schizophrenia 20 years later. In: Häffler H, Gattaz WF, Janzarik W, eds. *Search for the Cause of Schizophrenia.* Springer-Verlag: Berlin Heidelberg; 223-235.

91. Olney JW, Newcomer JW, Farber BB. (1999). NMDA receptor hypofunction model of schizophrenia. *Journal of Psychiatric Research,* 33, 523-533.

92. Javitt DC, Zukin SR. (1991). Recent advances in the phencyclidine model of schizophrenia *Am J Psychiatry.* 148:1301-1308.

93. Lane HY, Chang YC, Liu YC, Chiu CC, Tsai GE. (2005). Sarcosine or D-serine add-on treatment for acute exacerbation of schizophrenia—a randomized, double-blind, placebo-controlled study. *Arch Gen Psychiatry.* 62:1196-1204.

94. Mahadik SP, Mukherjee S. (1996). Free radical pathology and antioxidant defense in schizophrenia: a review. *Schizophr Res.* 19:1-17.

95. Tosic M, Ott J, Barral S, et al. (2006). Schizophrenia and oxidative stress: glutamate cysteine ligase modifier as a susceptibility gene. *Am J Hum Genet.* 79(3):586-592.

96. Liebermann JA. (1999). Is schizophrenia a neurodegenerative disorder? A clinical and neurobiological perspective. *Biol Psychiatry.* 46(6):729-739.

97. Gottesman II, Shields J, Hanson DR. (1982). *Schizophrenia—The Epigenetic Puzzle.* Cambridge University Press. Cambridge, UK.

98. Petronis A, Paterson AD, Kennedy JL. (1999). Schizophrenia: An Epigenetic Puzzle? *Schizophr Bull.* 1999;25(4):639-655.

99. Freedman R, Adler LE, Leonard S. (1999). Alternative phenotypes for the complex genetics of schizophrenia. *Biol Psychiatry.* 45(5):551-558.

100. Petronis A, Gottesman II, Peixiang K, et al. (2003). Monozygotic twins exhibit numerous epigenetic differences: clues to twin discordance? *Schizophr Bull.* 29(1):169-178.

101. Kundakovic M, Chen Y, Costa E, Grayson DR. (2007). DNA methyltransferase inhibitors coordinately induce expression of the human reelin and GAD67 genes. *Mol Pharmacol.* 71:644-653.

102. Waltrip RW, Carrigan DR, Carpenter WT. (1990). Immunopathology and viral reactivation. A general theory of schizophrenia. *J Nerv Ment Dis.* 178(12):729-738.

103. Lane N. Born to the purple: the story of porphyria. (2002, December 16). *Sci Am.*

104. López-Muñoz F, Bhatara VS, Alamo C. (2004). Historical approach to reserpine discovery and its introduction in psychiatry. *Actas Esp Psiquiatr.* 32(6):387-395.

105. Schatzberg AF, Nemeroff CB. (2009). *Textbook of Psychopharmacology.* American Psychiatric Publishing, Inc.: Arlington VA.

106. Hirschfeld RM. (2000). History and evolution of the monoamine hypothesis of depression. *J Clin Psychiatry.* 61(suppl 6):4-6.

107. *Physician's Desk Reference 2010.* Thompson PDR: Montvale, NJ.

108. Fava M, Borus, JS, Alpert JE, Nierenberg AA, Rosenbaum JF, Bottiglieri T. (1997). Folate, vitamin B12, and homocysteine in major depressive disorder. *Am J Psychiatry.* 154(3):426-428.

109. Larkin RW. (2007). *Comprehending Columbine.* Temple University Press: Philadelphia.

110. Brewer GJ. (2000). Recognition, diagnosis, and management of Wilson's disease. *Proc Soc Exp Biol Med.* 223(1)39-46.

111. Crayton JW, Walsh WJ. (2007). Elevated serum copper levels in women with a history of post-partum depression. *J Trace Elements Med Biol.* 21:17-21.

112. Klassen CD. (1996). *Casarett & Doull's Toxicology, the Basic Science of Poisons.* 5th ed. McGraw-Hill: New York.

113. Kanner L. (1943). Autistic disturbances of affective contact. *Nerv Child.* 2:217-250.

114. Kanner L, ed. (1973). *Childhood Psychosis: Initial Studies and New Insights.* V. H. Winston: Washington, DC.

115. Monitoring network, United States, 2006. (2006). *MMWR Surveillance Summaries.* Centers for Disease Control and Prevention: Washington, DC.

116. Freitag CM. (2007). The genetics of autistic disorders and its clinical relevance: a review of the literature. *Mol Psychiatry.* 12(1):2-22.

117. Stefanatos GA. (2008). Regression in autistic spectrum disorders. *Neuropsychol Rev.* 18(4):305-319.

118. Bettelheim B. (1967). *The Empty Fortress: Infantile Autism and the Birth of the Self.* The Free Press: New York.

119. Walsh WJ, Usman A, Tarpey J. Disordered metal metabolism in a large autism population. *Proceedings of the American Psychiatric Association.* New Research: Abstract NR109; May 9, 2001, New Orleans, LA.

120. Dziobek I, Bahnermann M, Convit A, Heekeren HR. (2010). The role of the fusiform-amygdala system in the pathophysiology of autism. *Arch Gen Psychiatry.* 67(4)397-405.

121. Kemper TL, Baumann M. (1998). Neuropathology of infantile autism. *J Neuropathol Exp Neurol.* 57:645-652.

122. Bauman ML, Kemper TL. (2005). Neuroanatomic observations of the brain in autism. *Int J Dev Neurosci.* 23:183-187.

123. Casanova MF. (2004). White matter increase and minicolumns in autism. *Ann Neurol.* 56:453.

124. Casanova MF, Buxhoeveden D, Switala A, Roy E. (2002). Minicolumnar pathology in autism. *Neurology.* 58:428-432.

125. Evans TA, Siedlak SL, Lu L, McGinnis W, Walsh W, et al. (2008). The autistic phenotype exhibits a remarkably localized modification of brain protein by products of free radical-induced lipid oxidation. *Am J Biochem Biotech.* 4(2):61-72.

126. Courchesne E, Carper R, Akshoomoof N. (2003). Evidence of brain overgrowth in the first year of life in autism. *JAMA.* 290(3):337-344.

127. Vargas DL, Nascimbene C, Krishnan C, Zimmerman AW, Pardo CA. (2005). Neuroglial activation and neuroinflammation in the brain of patients with autism. *Ann Neurol.* 55(2):257-267.

128. Pangborn J, Baker SM. (2005). *Autism: Effective Biomedical Treatments.* Autism Research Institute: San Diego, CA.

129. Russo AJ. (2009). Decreased serum Cu/Zn SOD in children with autism. *Nutr Metab Insights.* 2:27-35.

130. Keenan M, Henderson M, Kerr KP, Dillenburger K, eds.. (2005). *Applied Behaviour Analysis And Autism: Building a Future Together.* Jessica Kingsley Publishers: London.

131. Kearney AJ. (2007). *Understanding Applied Behavior Anaylsis: An Introduction to ABA for Parents, Teachers, and Other Professionals.* Jessica Kingsley Publishers: London.

132. Barbera M, Rasmussen T. (2007). *The Verbal Behavior Approach: How to Teach Children with Autism and Related Disorders.* Jessica Kingsley Publishers: London.

133. Hibbs ED, Jensen PS, eds. (2005). *Psychosocial Treatments for Child and Adolescent Disorders: Empirically Based Strategies for Clinical Practice.* 2nd ed. American Psychological Association: Washington, DC.

134. Cooper JO, Heron TE, Heward WL. (2007). *Applied Behavior Analysis.* 2nd ed. Prentice Hall: Upper Saddle River, NJ.

135. Simpson RL. (1999). Early Intervention with Children with Autism: The Search for Best Practices. *J Assoc Persons with Severe Handicaps.* 24(3):218-221.

136. US Department of Health & Human Services. (1999). *Mental Health: A Report of the Surgeon General—Executive Summary.* US Department of Health & Human Services, Substance Abuse and Mental Health Services Administration, Center for Mental Health Services, National Institutes of Health, National Institute of Mental Health: Rockville, MD.

137. Pardo CA, Vargas DL, Zimmerman AW. (2005). Immunity, neuroglia and neuroinflammation in autism. *Int Rev Psychiatry.* 17(6):485.

138. Reichelt KL, Knivsberg A-M, Lind G, Nødland M. (1991). Probable etiology and possible treatment of childhood autism. *Brain Dysfunct.* 4:308-319.

139. Jain KK. (1996). *Textbook of Hyperbaric Medicine.* 2nd ed. Hogrefe and Huber Publishers, Inc.: Cambridge, MA.

140. Walsh W (2012). Risperdal and brain shrinkage: a warning for autism families. *Autism Science Digest.* 4:128.

141. McCracken JT, McGough J, Shah B. (2002). Risperidone in children with autism and serious behavioral problems. *NEJM.* 347:314-321.

142. Dorph-Peterson K-A, Pierri JN, Sun Z, Sampson AR, Lewis DA (2005). The influence of chronic exposure to antipsychotic medications on brain size before and after tissue fixation: a comparison of haloperidol and olanzapine in macaque monkeys. *Neuropsycopharmacology.* 30(9): 1649-61.

143. Konopaske GT, Dorph-Peterson K-A, Pierri JN, Wu Q, Sampson AR, Lewis DA (2007). Effect of chronic exposure to antipsychotic medications on cell numbers in the parietal cortex of macaque monkeys. *Neuropsychopharmacology.* 32(6): 1216-23.

144. Konopaske GT, Dorph-Peterson K-A, Sweet RA, Pierri JN, Zhang W, Sampson AR, Lewis DA (2008). Effect of chronic antipsychotic exposure on astrocyte and oligodendrocyte numbers in macaque monkeys. *Biol Psychiatry.* 63(8): 759-765.

145. Harrison PJ, Lewis DA (2003). Neuropathology of schizophrenia. In: Hirsch S, Weinberger DR, eds. *Schizophrenia.* 2nd ed. Oxford, England: Blackwell Science Ltd (310-325).

146. Lewis DA (2011). Antipsychotic medications and brain volume. Do we have cause for concern? (Editorial). *Arch Gen Psych*, 68(2): 126-7.

147. Walsh WJ, Usman AL, inventors. Nutrient Supplements and Methods for Treating Autism and for Preventing the Onset of Autism. US Patent No. 7,232,575; June 19, 2007.

148. Stromland K, Nordin V, Miller M, Akerstrom B, Gilberg C. (1994). Autism in thalidomide embryopathy: a population study. *Dev Med Child Neurol.* 36(4):351-356.

149. Tost J. (2008). *Epigenetics.* Chapter 16 (371-376). Caister Academic Press: Norfolk, UK.

150. Walsh WJ, Glab LB, Haakenson ML. (2004). Reduced violent behavior following biochemical therapy. *Physiol Behav.* 82:835-839.

151. Wilson JQ, Herrnstein RJ. (1985). *Crime and human nature.* New York: Simon and Schuster.

152. Graeber MB, Mehraein P. (1999). Reanalysis of the first case of Alzheimer's disease. *Eur Arch Psychiatry Clin Neurosci.* 249(suppl 3):10-13.

153. Kraepelin E. (1910). Psychiatrie: Ein Lehrbuch fur Studierende und Arzte. *Leipzig: Barth.* 1910:593-632.

154. Folstein MF, Folstein SE, McHugh PR. (1975). Mini-mental state. A practical method for grading the cognitive state of patients for the clinician. *J Psychiatric Res.* 12(3):189-198.

155. Robbins TW, James M, Owen AM, Sahakian BJ, McInnes L, Rabbitt P. (1994). Cambridge Neuropsychological Test Automated Battery (CANTAB): a factor analytic study of a large sample of normal elderly volunteers. *Dementia.* 5(5):266-281.

156. Hoyert DL, Rosenberg HM. (1997). Alzheimer's disease as a cause of death in the United States. *Public Health Rep.* 112(6):497-505.

157. Campion D, Brice A, Hannequin D, et al. (1995). A large pedigree with early-onset Alzheimer's disease: clinical, neuropathologic, and genetic characterization. *Neurology.* 45(1):80-85.

158. Saunders AM, Schmader K, Breitner JCS, et al. (1993). Apolipoprotein E epsilon 4 allele distributions in late-onset Alzheimer's disease and in other amyloid-forming diseases. *Lancet.* 342:710-711.

159. Katzman R, Bick K. (2000). *Alzheimer Disease: The Changing View.* Academic Press: London.

160. Plassman BL, Havlik RJ, Steffens DC, et al. (2000). Documented head injury in early adulthood and risk of Alzheimer's disease and other dementias. *Neurology.* 55(8):1158-1166.

161. Roberts AH. (1969). *Brain Damage in Boxers*. Pitman Medical Scientific Publishing Co.: London.

162. Roe CM, Mintun MA, D'Angelo G, Xiong C, Grant EA, Morris JC. (2008). Alzheimer's disease and cognitive reserve. *Arch Neurol.* 65(11):1467-1471.

163. Scarmeas N. (2006). Education and rates of cognitive decline in incident Alzheimer's disease. *J Neurol Neurosurg Psychiatry.* 77:308-316.

164. Wilson RS, Mendes de Leon CF, Barnes LI, et al. Participation in cognitively stimulating activities and risk of incident Alzheimer disease. *JAMA.* Feb 13, 2002.

165. Larson EB. (2008). Physical activity for older adults at risk for Alzheimer disease. *JAMA.* 300(9):1077-1079.

166. Mielke MM, Rosenberg PB, Tschanz J, et al. (2007). Vascular factors predict rate of progression in Alzheimer disease. *Neurology.* 69:1850-1858.

167. Truelsen T, Thudium D, Gronbaek M. (2002). Amount and type of alcohol and risk of dementia: The Copenhagen Heart Study. *Neurology.* 59:1313-1319.

168. Mruthinti S, Schade RF, Harrell DU, et al. (2006). Autoimmunity in Alzheimer's Disease as evidenced by plasma immunoreactivity against RAGE and Aβ42: complication of diabetes. *Curr Alzheimer Res.* 3(3):229-235.

169. Cornett CR, Markesbery WR, Ehmann WD. (1998). Imbalances of trace elements related to oxidative damage in Alzheimer's disease brain. *Neurotoxicity.* 19:339-346.

170. Solfrizzi V, Panza F, Capurso A. (2003). The role of diet in cognitive decline. *J Neural Trans.* 110:95-110.

171. Seshadri S, Beiser A, Selhub J, et al. (2002). Plasma homocysteine as a risk factor for dementia and Alzheimer's disease. *NEJM.* 346:476-483.

172. Boiler F, Forette F. (1989). Alzheimer's disease and THA: a review of the cholinergic theory and of preliminary results. *Biomed Pharmacother.* 43(7):487-491.

173. Davis KL, Mohs RC, Marin D, et al. (1999). Cholinergic markers in elderly patients with early signs of Alzheimer disease. *JAMA.* 281(15):1401-1406.

174. Shankar GM, Li S, Mehta TH, et al. (2008). Amyloid-beta protein dimers isolated directly from Alzheimer's brains impair synaptic plasticity and memory. *Nat Med.* 14(8):837-842.

175. Hartmann T, Bieger SC, Brühl B, et al. (1997). Distinct sites of intracellular production for Alzheimer's disease A beta40/42 amyloid peptides. *Nat Med.* 3(9):1016-1020.

176. Schenk D, Barbour R, Dunn W, et al. (1999). Immunization with amyloid-beta attenuates Alzheimer-disease-like pathology in the PDAPP mouse. *Nature.* 400:173-177.

177. Town T. (2009). Alternative Aβ immunotherapy approaches for Alzheimer's disease. *CNS Neurol Disord Drug Targets.* 8(2):114-127.

178. Blennow K, Wallin A, Agren H, Spenger C, Siegfried J, Vanmechelen E. (1995). Tau protein in cerebrospinal fluid: a biochemical marker for axonal degeneration in Alzheimer disease? *Mol Chem Neuropathol.* 26(3)231-245.

179. Zhang Q, Powers ET, Nieva J, et al. (2004). Metabolite-initiated protein misfolding may trigger Alzheimer's disease. *Proc Natl Acad Sci.* 101(14):4752-4757.

180. Markesbery WR. (1997). Oxidative stress hypothesis in Alzheimer's disease. *Free Radic Biol Med.* 23(1):134-147.

181. Perry G, Cash AD, Smith MA. (2002). *Alzheimer disease and oxidative stress. J Biomed Biotechnol.* 2(3):120-123.

182. Lee HP, Zhu X, Casadesus G, et al. (2010). Antioxidant approaches for the treatment of Alzheimer's disease. *Expert Rev Neurother.* 10(7):1201-1208.

183. Hung YH, Bush AI, Cherny RA. (2010). Copper in the brain and Alzheimer's disease. *J Biol Inorg Chem.* 15(1):61-76.

184. House E, Mold M, Collingwood J, Baldwin A, Goodwin S, Exley C. (2009). Copper Abolishes the β-Sheet Secondary Structure of Preformed Amyloid Fibrils of Amyloid-β. *J Alzheimer's Dis.* 18:811-817.

185. Yang XH, Huang HC, Chen L, Xu W, Jiang ZF. (2009). Coordinating to three histidine residues: Cu(II) promotes oligomeric and fibrillar amyloid-β peptide to precipitate in a non-β aggregation way. *J Alzheimer's Dis.* 18(4):799-810.

186. Walsh WJ, Lai B, Bazan N, Lukiw WL. (March 1, 2005). Trace metal analysis in Alzheimer's disease tissues using high-brilliance x-ray beams. *Proceedings of the 6th Keele Meeting on Trace Metals and Neurotoxicity in the Brain.* Portugal.

187. Yu WH, Lukiw WJ, Bergeron C, Niznik HB, Fraser PE. (2001). Metallothionein III is reduced in Alzheimer's disease. *Brain Res.* 894(1):37-45.

188. Uchida Y, Takio K, Titani K, Ihara Y, Tomonaga M. (1991). The growth inhibitory factor that is deficient in the Alzheimer's-disease brain is a 68-amino acid metallothionein-like protein. *Neuron.* 7(2):337-347.

189. LaRowe SD, Myrick H, Kalivas PW, et al. (2007). Is cocaine desire reduced by N-acetylcysteine? *Am J Psychiatry.* 164:1115-1117.

190. Vengeliene V, Kiefer F, Spanagel R. (2011). D-cycloserine facilitates extinction of alcohol-seeking behavior in rats. *Alcohol and Alcoholism.* 43(6):626-629.

191. Lovinger DM, White G, Weight FF. (1989). Ethanol inhibits NMDA-activated ion current in hippocampal neurons. *Science.* 243(4899):1721-1724.

GLOSSARY

Acetyl coenzyme A: An important molecule in metabolism that is involved in many biochemical reactions. It is the primary source of acetyl groups for epigenetic histone modification, synthesis of the neurotransmitter acetylcholine, and fat metabolism.

Acetyl groups: In organic chemistry, acetyl is a functional group with the chemical formula $COCH_3$. The acetyl group consists of a methyl group single-bonded to a carbonyl.

Acetyltransferases: Enzymes that transfer an acetyl group to a histone or another protein.

Acetylcholine: A monoamine neurotransmitter essential to memory, communication between nerves and muscles, and parasympathetic activity.

Adrenochrome theory: A hypothesis that schizophrenics lack the ability to remove the hallucinogenic metabolite adrenochrome from their brains.

Albumin: The main protein of plasma; it binds water, cations (such as Ca^{++}, Na^{+} and K^{+}), fatty acids, hormones, bilirubin, and drugs—its main function is to regulate the osmotic pressure of blood.

Aldehyde: An organic compound with the structure R-CHO, consisting of a carbonyl center bonded to hydrogen and an R group.

Alkaline (basic): The opposite of acidic, with pH level above 7.0.

Allele: One of a group of genes that occur alternatively at a specific DNA location.

Alzheimer's disease (AD): A progressive and fatal brain disease that destroys brain cells, causing memory loss and problems with thinking and behavior.

Amygdala: Almond-shaped structures located deep within the medial temporal lobes of the brain that are essential to memory and emotional reaction and are considered part of the limbic system.

Amygdala-fusiform system: A brain location containing the amygdala and fusiform gyrus.

Amenorrhea: The absence of a menstrual period in a woman of reproductive age.

Amino acid: A molecule containing an amine group, a carboxylic acid group, and a side chain that varies among different amino acids. Amino acids are critical to life and have many functions in metabolism including the formation of proteins, enzymes, cofactors, and other biochemicals.

Amphetamine: A psychostimulant drug known to produce increased wakefulness and focus in association with decreased fatigue and appetite. Amphetamines are believed to act by increasing synaptic activities of dopamine and norepinephrine in the brain. Popular amphetamines include Ritalin and Adderal.

Amyloid plaque: A "sticky" buildup of deviant amyloid protein that accumulates outside brain cells in Alzheimer's disease.

Angiogenesis: The physiological process involving the growth of new blood vessels from pre-existing vessels.

Anorexia nervosa: An eating disorder characterized by refusal to maintain a healthy body weight and an obsessive fear of gaining weight due to a distorted self image. It is a serious mental illness with a high incidence of comorbidity and has the highest mortality rate of any psychiatric disorder.

Antidepressant: A psychiatric medication used to alleviate mood disorders, such as major depression, dysthymia, and anxiety disorders. This family of drugs includes monoamine oxidase inhibitors (MAOIs), tricyclic antidepressants (TCAs), selective serotonin reuptake inhibitors (SSRIs), and serotonin-norepinephrine reuptake inhibitors (SNRIs).

Antioxidant: A molecule capable of inhibiting the oxidation of other molecules. Antioxidants can protect the body against formation of free radicals that can damage cells.

Antisocial personality disorder (ASPD): A psychiatric condition in which a person manipulates, exploits, or violates the rights of others and may engage in criminal activity. Typical symptoms include stealing, narcissism, oppositional defiance, fighting, absence of remorse, and disregard for safety of self and others.

ApoE proteins: A class of proteins essential for the normal catabolism of triglyceride-rich lipoprotein constituents. Genetic ApoE variants (alleles) have an important role in determining the risk of Alzheimer's disease.

Applied behavior analysis (ABA): A science in which the principles of behavior analysis are applied systematically to improve socially significant behavior. It is a popular treatment for children diagnosed with an autism spectrum disorder.

Aspartic acid: An amino acid [$HO_2CCH(NH_2)CH_2CO_2H$] that serves as an excitatory neurotransmitter in the brain and is an excitotoxin.

Asperger's disorder (aka Asperger's syndrome): A developmental disorder on the autism spectrum that affects a child's ability to socialize and communicate effectively with others. Children with Asperger's syndrome typically exhibit social awkwardness and an all-absorbing interest in specific topics.

Atherosclerosis: The build-up of a waxy plaque on the inside of blood vessels sometimes referred to as hardening of the arteries.

Atrial fibrillation: A heart disorder in which the two upper chambers beat chaotically and irregularly—out of coordination with the two lower chambers (the ventricles) of the heart. Symptoms include an irregular and often rapid heart rate, palpitations, shortness of breath, and weakness.

Attention-deficit/hyperactivity disorder (ADHD): A neurobehavioral developmental disorder that can be a barrier to academic and career success. Primary symptoms usually include high physical activity, inattentiveness, and impulsivity.

Atypical antipsychotic medications: A group of antipsychotic tranquilizing drugs used to treat psychiatric conditions including schizophrenia, mania, and bipolar disorder by blocking receptors in the brain's dopamine pathways.

Autism spectrum disorder (ASD): A severe disorder of neural development characterized by impaired social interaction and communication and by restricted and repetitive behaviors. Autism affects information processing in the brain by altering how nerve cells and their synapses connect and organize, with onset by age 3.

Axon: A long, slender projection of a nerve cell, or neuron, that conducts electrical impulses away from the neuron's cell body or soma.

Benzodiazapine: A class of psychoactive drugs whose core chemical structure is the fusion of a benzene ring and a diazepine ring. Benzodiazepines enhance the effect of the neurotransmitter GABA, which generally results in sedation, reduced anxiety, and improved ability to sleep.

Bipolar disorder: A serious psychiatric condition that usually involves episodes of abnormally elevated energy levels, cognition, and mood (mania) followed by episodes of clinical depression. The disorder has been subdivided into bipolar I, bipolar II, cyclothymia, and other types, based on the nature and severity of mood episodes experienced; the range is often described as the bipolar spectrum.

Biochemical: An atom or molecule intrinsic to the body that participates in chemical processes in the body. There are a vast number of biochemicals in humans, including proteins, enzymes, nutrients, fatty acids, and hormones. An example of what we refer to as a biochemical is vitamin B-6 as well as its derivative pyridoxal-5'-phosphate (PLP).

Biochemical individuality: The concept that the nutritional and chemical make-up of each person is unique and that dietary needs, therefore, vary from person to person.

Biochemical therapy: Medical treatments that use natural body chemicals rather than drugs.

Biotype: A group of persons who share specific biochemical factors.

Blood-brain barrier (BBB): High-density cells attached to blood vessels that prevent or restrict the passage of certain chemicals into the brain.

Brain bank: An organized collection and storage of postmortem brains for the purpose of scientific research. Most brain banks are dedicated to studies of specific disorders such as autism, Alzheimer's disease, etc.

Brush border: A high-area section of the intestines (or kidneys) containing microvilli that enable rapid and efficient transport of nutrients (or wastes).

Bulemia: An eating disorder characterized by recurrent binge eating, followed by compensatory behaviors such as vomiting (or purging), use of laxatives, enemas, etc

Cambridge Neuropsychological Test Automated Battery (CANTAB): A computer-based cognitive assessment system consisting of a battery of neuropsychological tests, administered to subjects using a touch screen computer.

Carboxyethylpyrrole: An organic chemical that results from free-radical induced oxidation of the essential fatty acid DHA.

Carboxyl group: A functional group consisting of a carbonyl and a hydroxyl, which has the formula of $-C(=O)OH$, usually written as $-COOH$ or $-CO_2H$.

Casomorphin: Protein fragments derived from incomplete digestion of milk protein, believed by many to have an opioid effect.

Catalase: An antioxidant enzyme that catalyzes the decomposition of hydrogen peroxide to water and oxygen.

Catatonia: A symptom of schizophrenia characterized by stupor or mutism, negativism, rigidity, purposeless excitement, and inappropriate or bizarre posturing.

Cerebellum: A region of the brain that has the appearance of a separate structure beneath the hemispheres. It plays an important role in motor control, the ability to have smooth physical movements, and cognitive functions such as attention and language.

Ceruloplasmin: The major copper-carrying protein in the blood, which also plays a role in iron metabolism.

Chelation therapy: The administration of oral or intravenous chemicals to remove heavy metals from the body.

Cholinergic: An adjective used to describe enhancement of acetylcholine activity in the brain and the peripheral nervous system.

Chromatin: The combination of DNA and proteins that makes up chromosomes. The major components are DNA and histone proteins, although other proteins have prominent roles too. The functions of chromatin are to package DNA into a smaller volume to fit in the cell nucleus, to strengthen the DNA to allow mitosis and meiosis, and to regulate gene expression and DNA replication.

Crohn's disease: A form of inflammatory bowel disease (IBD) that usually affects the intestines but may occur anywhere from the mouth to the end of the rectum (anus).

Citrulline: A protein made from ornithine and carbamoyl phosphate in one of the central reactions in the urea cycle. It is sometimes used for the purpose of athletic enhancement.

Coenzyme: A small organic molecule that links to an enzyme and whose presence is essential to the activity of that enzyme.

Cofactor: A nonprotein chemical that is loosely bound to a protein (or enzyme) and is required for the protein's biological activity.

Conduct disorder (CD): A psychiatric condition marked by a pattern of repetitive violation of the rights of others. Symptoms include verbal and physical aggression, cruel behavior toward people and pets, destructive behavior, lying, truancy, vandalism, and stealing.

Controlled study: A clinical study that compares people getting treatment (treatment group) to persons who do not receive this treatment (control group).

Coproporphyria (aka hereditary coproporphyria or HCP): A form of hepatic porphyria associated with a deficiency of the enzyme coproporphyrinogen III oxidase.

Cortex: The cerebrum or cortex is the largest part of the human brain, associated with higher brain functions such as thought and action. The cerebral cortex is divided into four sections, called lobes: frontal lobe, parietal lobe, occipital lobe, and temporal lobe.

CpG islands: Genomic regions that contain a high frequency of cytosine-phosphate-guanine sites.

Creatine: A nitrogenous organic acid that occurs naturally in humans and helps to supply energy to muscle. It is commonly used by athletes to enhance physical endurance.

Cyclothymic disorder: A mild form of bipolar disorder in which a person has mood swings ranging from mild-to-moderate depression to euphoria and excitement but stays connected to reality.

Cystathionine beta-synthase (aka cystathionine β-synthase or CBS): The enzyme that converts homocysteine to cystathionine.

Cystathionine pathway: Conversion of homocysteine to cystathionine, which in turn reacts to produce cysteine, glutathione, and other important sulfur proteins.

Cytosol: A complex mixture of substances dissolved in water that forms the fluid within cells.

Deacetylases: A class of enzymes that remove acetyl groups from molecules. Its action is opposite to that of an acetyltransferase.

Delusional disorder: A psychotic mental disorder involving non-bizarre delusions in the absence of any other significant form of psychosis. These persons have fixed beliefs that are certainly and definitely false but are somewhat plausible, for example, someone who thinks he or she is being followed by the CIA.

Dementia praecox: An obsolete psychiatric diagnosis developed in the 19th century to describe a chronic, deteriorating psychotic disorder characterized by rapid cognitive disintegration, usually beginning in the late teens or early adulthood.

Depression: A mental disorder characterized by a pervasive low mood, usually accompanied by low self-esteem and by loss of interest or pleasure in normally enjoyable activities.

Dendrites: The branched projections of a neuron that conduct electrochemical signals from other neural cells to the cell body of the neuron from which the dendrites project.

Dismutase: An antioxidant enzyme that converts superoxide (O_2-) free radicals to a less aggressive molecule, H_2O_2.

DNA: Deoxyribonucleic acid is a molecule that contains the genetic instructions used in the development and functioning of all living beings. DNA is often compared to a set of blueprints, since it contains the instructions needed to construct other cell components, such as proteins and RNA molecules. The DNA segments that carry this genetic information are called genes.

DNA methylation: A natural process in which parts of the DNA receive a methyl group that results in regulation of gene expression or inhibition. It is also one of the two epigenetic processes that can alter expression of specific genes.

DNA promoter region: A regulatory region of DNA located upstream of a gene, providing a control point for regulated gene transcription.

Dopamine beta-hydroxylase (aka dopamine β-hydroxylase or DBH): A copper-containing oxygenase enzyme that converts dopamine to norepinephrine.

Dopamine: A catecholamine neurotransmitter that is also a precursor of norepinephrine and adrenaline.

Dopamine transporter (DAT): A membrane-spanning protein that pumps the neurotransmitter dopamine out of the synapse back into the cytosol of dopamine cells for later storage and release.

Double-blind study: An experimental procedure in which neither the subjects of the experiment nor the persons administering the experiment know certain critical aspects of the experiment until the results have been recorded. This protocol guards against experimenter bias and enables measurement of placebo effects.

Double helix: In molecular biology, this term refers to the structure formed by double-stranded molecules of nucleic acids. The DNA double helix is a spiral polymer of nucleic acids, held together by nucleotides with the two DNA strands connected in multiple locations by hydrogen atoms to form base pairs.

DSM-IV-TR: *The Diagnostic and Statistical Manual of Mental Disorders, Fourth Edition, Text Revision,* published by the American Psychiatric Association.

Dysthemia: A mild but chronic form of depression.

Eczema: A chronic skin disorder that involves scaly and itchy rashes.

Enzyme: A protein (or conjugated protein) produced in the body that catalyzes or speeds up a chemical reaction.

Epigenetics: The study of changes in gene activity that do not involve alterations to the genetic code, especially DNA methylation and histone modification.

Epilepsy: A common chronic neurological disorder characterized by recurrent, unprovoked seizures, caused by episodic abnormal electrical activity in the brain.

Estrogen: A female hormone produced by the ovaries.

Exorcism: An ancient practice of driving out demons or evil spirits from persons, places, or things that are believed to be possessed or infested by them.

Folate: A water-soluble B vitamin that occurs naturally in food, necessary for the production and maintenance of new cells, for synthesis of DNA and RNA, and for preventing changes to DNA.

Forensics: The application of a broad spectrum of sciences to answer questions of interest to the legal system, especially in relation to a crime.

Free radical: An atom or molecule that has a single unpaired electron in an outer shell that can react with and damage biological structures.

Gamma-aminobutyric acid (aka γ-aminobutyric acid or GABA): The chief inhibitory (calming) neurotransmitter in the central nervous system.

Gene: A hereditary unit consisting of a sequence of DNA that occupies a specific location on a chromosome and determines a particular characteristic in an organism.

Genetics: The branch of biology that deals with heredity, especially the mechanisms of hereditary transmission and the variation of inherited characteristics among similar or related organisms.

Gene expression: The process by which information from a gene is used in the synthesis of a protein.

Genome: The entirety of an organism's hereditary information, including both the genes and the noncoding sequences of its DNA.

Glial cells: Nonneural cells that support neurons by providing physical support and nutrition and perform housekeeping functions such as clearing out debris and excess materials. Glial cells in the brain consist of astrocytes, oligodendrocytes, and microglia.

Gluteomorphin: Protein fragments derived from incomplete digestion of gluten protein, believed by many to have an opioid effect.

Gluten: The composite of two proteins called gliadin and glutenin found in some grass-related grains, notably wheat, rye, and barley.

Golgi apparatus: An organelle (or structure) found in the nucleus of a cell that processes proteins and fats produced in the reticulum and prepares them for export outside the nucleus.

Hallucination: A mistaken perception of visual, auditory, tactile, olfactory, or other sensory experience without an external stimulus and with a compelling sense of its reality, usually resulting from a mental disorder or as a response to a drug.

Hawthorne effect: Improvement or modification of an experimental subject's behavior, simply in response to the fact that they are being studied.

Heme: A chemical group consisting of an iron atom contained in the center of a large porphyrin ring that is a primary constituent of hemoglobin and other hemoproteins.

Hippocampus: A brain structure that lies under the medial temporal lobe, one on each side of the brain. It is critical for the formation of new memories and has an important role in learning and behavior.

Hirsutism: Excessive growth of body or facial hair.

Histadelia: A medical condition characterized by elevated levels of blood histamine.

Histamine: A physiologically active amine noted as $C_5H_9N_3$ that is found in plant and animal tissue and released from mast cells as part of an allergic reaction in humans. It stimulates gastric secretion, causes dilation of capillaries, constriction of bronchial smooth muscle, decreased blood pressure, and also functions as a neurotransmitter.

Histapenia: A medical condition characterized by low levels of blood histamine.

Histone: Histones are strongly alkaline proteins found in cell nuclei, which package DNA into structural units called nucleosomes. They are the chief protein components of chromatin, act as spools around which DNA winds, and play a role in gene regulation.

Histone modification: Epigenetic alteration of gene expression due to specific chemical reactions at histone tails.

Histone tails: Linear histone segments that protrude from the nucleosome that have an important role in regulating gene expression.

Homocysteine: An amino acid with the formula $HSCH_2CH_2CH(NH_2)CO_2H$. It is biosynthesized from methionine by the removal of its terminal C^ε methyl group.

Homocysteine can be recycled into methionine or converted into cysteine with the aid of B vitamins.

Homocysteinuria: Homocysteinuria, also known as cystathionine beta-synthase deficiency, is an inherited disorder of the metabolism of methionine. It involves an inherited autosomal recessive trait, with two copies of an autosomal gene -- one from each parent.

Hormone: A chemical released by a cell in one part of the body that sends out messages that affect cells in other parts of the body.

Hydroxyhemopyrrolin-2-one (HPL): A chemical in urine associated with elevated oxidative stress (mauve factor).

Hydroxyl group: An oxygen atom bound covalently with a hydrogen atom. The neutral form of this group is a hydroxyl radical. Organic molecules containing a hydroxyl group are known as alcohols.

Hyperactivity: A physical state in which a person is abnormally and easily excitable or exuberant, often resulting in strong emotional reactions, impulsive behavior, and a short attention span.

Hypercupremia: A metal metabolism disorder in which copper levels in blood and tissues may escalate to dangerous levels.

Immune function: A complex network of tissues, organs, cells, and chemicals that protects the body from infection and illness.

Inflammation: A localized protective reaction of tissue to irritation, injury, or infection, characterized by pain, redness, swelling, and sometimes loss of function.

Intermittent explosive disorder (IED): A behavioral disorder characterized by extreme expressions of anger, often to the point of uncontrollable rage, that are unpremeditated and disproportionate to the situation at hand.

Isoform: Any of two or more functionally similar proteins that have a similar but not identical amino acid sequence.

Learning disability: A neurological disorder in which a person has difficulty learning in a typical manner, usually involving the brain's ability to receive and process information.

L-Histadine: An essential amino acid from which histamine is derived.

Libido: Emotional or psychic energy derived from primitive biological urges, often associated with sex drive.

Lipid: A diverse group of naturally occurring molecules that includes fats, waxes, sterols, fat-soluble vitamins, monoglycerides, diglycerides, phospholipids, and others. Lipids are the primary constituents of cell membranes and have a role in energy storage.

Lysergic acid diethylamide (LSD): Colloquially known as acid, LSD is a psychedelic drug of the ergoline family and a nonaddictive recreational drug known for its psychological effects, which can include altered thinking processes, time distortion, and a sense of having a spiritual experience.

Malabsorption: Faulty absorption of nutrient materials from the alimentary canal.

Monoamine oxidase inhibitor (MAOI): An antidepressant medication that elevates serotonin activity by blocking monoamine oxidase, an enzyme that metabolizes (destroys) serotonin.

Mauve factor: A chemical in urine associated with elevated oxidative stress: hydroxy-hemopyrrolin-2-one (HPL).

Melancholia: A mental condition characterized by extreme depression, bodily complaints, and often hallucinations and delusions.

Mendelian genetics: The laws of inheritance relating to the transmission of hereditary characteristics from parents to their offspring.

Metabolic syndrome: A potentially fatal syndrome involving high blood pressure, obesity, high cholesterol, and insulin resistance; a dangerous side effect of many antipsychotic medications.

Metallothionein: A family of four low-molecular-weight, cysteine-rich proteins that have potent metal binding and redox capabilities and are involved in early brain development. They have powerful antioxidant properties and work together with glutathione and selenium to protect against toxic metals.

Methyl group: A reactive chemical entity with formula CH_3^- that participates in many dozens of biochemical reactions.

Methylation: The addition of a methyl group to a molecule or atom, which is a primary factor in epigenetic modification of gene expression.

Methylenetetrahydrofolate reductase (MTHFR) enzyme: An important enzyme that plays a role in processing proteins and regulating methyl levels.

Micron: A unit of distance equal to one-millionth of a meter.

Microtubules: Components of brain cells that provide structural support for the axon, serve as a conduit for nutrients and organelles, and participate in cellular processes including mitosis. They are generally straight and about 24 nanometers in diameter.

Minicolumn: A vertical column of 80-120 brain neurons in the brain's cortex that are believed to act in concert. The estimated 200 million minicolumns in the adult brain are believed to have a strong role in brain organization and development.

Mini-mental test: The mini-mental state examination (MMSE) or Folstein test is a brief 30-point questionnaire used to screen for cognitive impairment. It is commonly used in medicine to assist in diagnosis for Alzheimer's disease and other forms of dementia.

Molecular biology: The study of biology at a molecular level, including the molecular nature of DNA, RNA, and the mechanisms of gene replication, mutation, and expression. This field combines the sciences of biology and chemistry and studies the mechanisms and kinetics of cellular and tissue processes.

Monoamine: A small molecule neurotransmitter that contains one amino group connected to an aromatic ring by a two-carbon chain ($-CH_2-CH_2-$). Examples include serotonin, dopamine, norepinephrine, epinephrine, histamine, and melatonin.

Monoamine oxidase: A family of enzymes that oxidize (break down) neurotransmitters at the synapse, reducing the population of those neurotransmitters and lowering synaptic activity.

Myelin: A structure of lipid fats and proteins that forms a sheath around the axons of neurons. Myelin provides electrical insulation and physical support for the cell and facilitates the transmission of nerve signals down the axon.

N-methyl-D-aspartate (NMDA) receptor: A complex type of glutamate receptor that requires activation by both glutamate and the amino acid glycine. It is believed to have a major role in schizophrenia and also in the development of learning and memory.

Nanogram: A unit of mass equal to 0.001 micrograms.

Negative symptoms of schizophrenia: Functional impairments often present in schizophrenia, including low motivation, reduced energy, social withdrawal, and impaired cognition. These are contrasted with symptoms such as hallucinations, paranoia, delusions, anxiety, and depression that are called "positive symptoms" in the psychiatry field.

Neurobiology (aka neuroscience): The study of molecular, developmental, structural, functional, and medical aspects of the nervous system.

Neurochemistry: The study of neurochemicals, which include neurotransmitters, psychiatric drugs, and other molecules that influence brain function.

Neurodegeneration: The progressive loss of structure or function of brain cells, usually involving death of the cells (apoptosis).

Neuron: An electrically excitable nerve cell that processes and transmits information by electrical and chemical signaling to other neurons across a synapse. Neurons interact with each other to form networks and are the core components of the brain and peripheral nervous system.

Neurotransmitter: A chemical that is released from a nerve cell (neuron) and transmits an impulse to another nerve cell. A neurotransmitter is a messenger of neurologic information from one cell to another. More than 100 neurotransmitters have been identified, including monoamines, amino acids, peptides, and other chemicals such as acetylcholine, zinc, and nitric oxide.

Norepinephrine: A catecholamine neurotransmitter synthesized from dopamine that also functions as a stress hormone. Elevated levels have been related to anxiety and panic disorders, and depressed levels have been related to catatonic tendencies.

Nucleosome: The basic unit of DNA packaging, consisting of a segment of DNA wound around a histone protein core.

Nutrient: A nourishing food substance that provides energy or is necessary for growth and repair. Examples of nutrients are vitamins, minerals, carbohydrates, fats, and proteins.

Obsessive-compulsive disorder (OCD): A mental disorder characterized by the presence of recurrent ideas and fantasies (obsessions), repetitive impulses or actions (compulsions), and high anxiety.

One-carbon cycle: A chemical cycle in which (a) dietary protein (methionine) is converted to a molecule (SAMe) that readily donates methyl groups for various reactions in the body, and in which (b) methionine levels are conserved by a series of chemical reactions.

Open-label study: A type of clinical trial in which both the researchers and participants know which treatment is being administered.

Oppositional defiant disorder (ODD): A behavioral disorder involving a pattern of disobedient, hostile, and defiant behavior toward authority figures.

Oxidative stress: A condition of increased oxidant production characterized by the excessive release of free radicals that can destroy cells or impair biochemical processes.

Paranoia: A psychological disorder characterized by delusions of persecution or grandeur.

Paranoid schizophrenia: A type of schizophrenia that involves psychosis (a departure from reality). It usually emerges during late teens or early adulthood and may involve delusions, auditory hallucinations, paranoia, depression, and high anxiety.

Paraphilias: A family of mental disorders involving recurrent and intense sexually arousing fantasies, urges, or behaviors of a peculiar or atypical nature. Included in this classification are pedophilia, exhibitionism, fetishism, frotteurism, sexual masochism, sexual sadism, and voyeurism. .

Parkinson's disease: A progressive disorder of the central nervous system associated with the degeneration of dopamine neurons in the *substantia nigra* area of the brain. Common symptoms are high-frequency tremors, muscle rigidity, slowed physical movements, an abnormal gait, impaired speech, and loss of facial expressions.

Parvalbumin: A calcium-binding albumin protein present in GABAergic neurons that modulates neuronal excitability and activity and is believed to have a strong role regarding inhibition of undesirable brain activity.

Pervasive developmental disorder—not otherwise specified (PDD-NOS): A diagnosis considered by many to represent a mild version of autism. Common symptoms include socialization deficits, repetitive behaviors, oversensitivity to certain visual stimuli, poor eye contact, speech problems, and difficulty making transitions.

Peptide: Any compound composed of a series of amino acids linked by covalent bonds. Peptide chains longer than a few dozen amino acids are usually called proteins. Many hormones, antibiotics, and other compounds that participate in life processes are peptides.

Phenocyclidine (PCP): A recreational drug of abuse known as angel dust that can produce hallucinations and neurotoxic effects.

Phenotype: A group or classification of persons sharing specific symptoms or characteristics.

Phlogiston theory: A mistaken belief originated by the ancient Greeks that fire involved a material called phlogiston that was released during combustion.

Phobia: An exaggerated and illogical fear of a particular object or class of objects.

Phosphate: Any of various salts or esters of phosphoric acid, characterized by a PO4 chemical group.

Photon beams: A concentrated and focused beam of radiant energy composed of light, gamma rays, or x-rays.

Pineal gland: A small endocrine gland in the brain that produces melatonin, a hormone that affects the modulation of wake/sleep patterns. This brain area is not protected by the blood-brain barrier.

Placebo effect: Improvement in the condition of an experimental subject that is not related to the treatment under study. The improvements may be due either to psychological expectations of benefits or changes in environment unknown to the experimenter.

Plaque: In biology, an extracellular protein buildup implicated in various diseases such as Alzheimer's disease.

Plasma: The fluid part of blood.

Polydypsia: An excessive water intake seen in some patients with a mental illness or a developmental disability.

Porphyria: A family of pathological states involving abnormalities of porphyrin metabolism, believed to be caused by disordered enzymes in the heme pathway.

Positive symptoms of schizophrenia: Hallucinations, paranoia, delusions, anxiety, depression, and other overt symptoms of schizophrenia. These are contrasted with the negative symptoms such as low motivation, reduced energy, social withdrawal, and impaired cognition.

Postpartum depression (PPD): Also known as postnatal depression, a form of clinical depression usually involving high anxiety that can affect women after childbirth.

Post-traumatic stress disorder (PTSD): A chronic anxiety disorder that can develop after exposure to a terrifying event in which grave physical harm occurred or was threatened, such as violent assaults, natural disasters, accidents, or military combat.

Presenilin proteins: A family of transmembrane proteins that play a key role in the modulation of intracellular Ca^{2+} involved in neurotransmitter release. Presenilin protein mutations have been implicated in early-onset Alzheimer's disease.

Presynaptic membrane: The part of the membrane of an axon terminal that faces the membrane of an adjacent brain cell across a synaptic gap and emits neurotransmitters that may activate the adjacent cell.

Presynaptic membrane protein: Specialized proteins in the vesicle wall, presynaptic membrane, and cytosol that assist vesicle docking, formation of a fusion pore, sensing of Ca^{++}, and neurotransmitter release.

Protein: A large molecule composed of one or more chains of amino acids in a specific order determined by the DNA coding for the protein. Proteins are required for the structure, function, and regulation of the body's cells, tissues, and organs.

Psychodynamic therapies: A psychiatric technique aimed at revealing the unconscious content of a client's psyche in an effort to alleviate psychic tension.

Psychosis: A symptom or feature of mental illness, usually characterized by radical changes in personality, impaired cognitive functioning, and a distorted sense of objective reality (hallucinations, delusions, paranoia, etc.).

Purkinje cells: Large brain neurons of the cerebral cortex having flask-shaped cell bodies with massive dendrites and one slender axon.

Pyridoxal-5'-phosphate (PLP or P-5-P): The active form of vitamin B6, which is produced in the body from pyridoxine hydrochloride and other forms of vitamin B-6 in the diet or nutritional supplements. It is available commercially as a nutritional supplement.

Pyrrole: A toxic liquid compound of composition C_4H_5N that has a ring consisting of four carbon atoms and one nitrogen atom, polymerizes readily in air, and is the parent compound of many biologically important substances, including bile pigments, porphyrins, and chlorophyll.

Radioimmune assay of hair (RIAH test): A laboratory assay for opiates, cocaine, PCP, and other drugs of abuse that can identify the timing and amount of drug usage for an individual.

Raphe nuclei: A moderate-sized cluster of neurons found in the brain stem that produce serotonin and release this neurotransmitter to the rest of the brain.

Receptor: A protein molecule, embedded in either the plasma membrane or the cytoplasm of a cell, that can receive a signal from a neurotransmitter or other signaling molecule.

Recommended dietary allowance (RDA): The daily amounts of protein, vitamins and minerals recommended by the government for healthy adults.

Regressive autism: A form of autism that appears abruptly after more than a year of typical childhood development, in which a child loses previously displayed skills, such as language and social skills.

Reticulum: A membrane cell component that receives RNA coding information, produces proteins, protects against certain toxic substances, and produces lipids.

Reuptake: A process by which a neurotransmitter in the synapse is returned to the original brain cell, usually facilitated by a special transmembrane transporter protein.

Ribonucleic acid (RNA): A single-stranded molecule transcribed from DNA that provides the genetic coding needed for production of specific proteins in the cell's reticulum.

Rumination: Excessive focus on past events, a common symptom of depression.

SAMe/SAH ratio: A useful laboratory blood test of a person's methylation status, involving assays for S-adenosylmethionine (SAMe) and S-adenosylhomocysteine (SAH).

Sarcosine: An amino acid derivative (N-methylglycine) believed to reduce symptoms of schizophrenia by enhancing glutamate activity at NMDA receptors.

Schizoaffective disorder: An adult-onset mental disorder usually characterized by deficits in cognition and emotion. Bizarre delusions, disorganized speech, and significant social and occupational dysfunction are common features of the disorder.

Schizophrenia: Any of several psychotic disorders that commonly involve auditory hallucinations, paranoid or bizarre delusions, disorganized speech, anxiety, depression, and other symptoms that usually result in significant social and occupational dysfunction.

Seasonal affective disorder (SAD): A type of depression that tends to occur at the same time every year.

Secretases: A family of enzymes believed responsible for creation of amyloid protein plaques in brain tissue (a pathological hallmark of Alzheimer's disease).

Selective serotonin reuptake inhibitor (SSRI): one of a family of antidepressant medications that inhibit the removal of serotonin from synapses by transport proteins (SERT).

Semaphorin: A family of transmembrane proteins that help growing axons find an appropriate target and also assist in formation of synapses.

Serotonin (5-HT): A monoamine neurotransmitter (5-Hydroxytryptamine) biochemically derived from tryptophan that has an important role in depression and other mental disorders.

Serotonin transporter (SERT): A special protein embedded in a presynaptic membrane that recycles serotonin transmitter molecules from a synapse back into the original cell.

Serum: The clear liquid that can be separated from clotted blood.

Sirtuins: A family of proteins that can remove acetyl groups (deacetylases) from histones thus tending to inhibit expression of a gene.

Spermine: A natural polyamine involved in cell metabolism that has a role in growth and stabilization of DNA structure.

Spleen: An organ that creates lymphocytes for the destruction and recycling of old red blood cells, acts as a blood reservoir, and assists in immune function.

Substantia nigra: A brain structure in the basal ganglia that is a primary site for dopamine activity and has a role in reward, movement, and addiction. Parkinson's disease results from the death of dopamine cells in the *substantia nigra*.

Superoxide dismutase (SOD): A natural metalloenzyme that provides important antioxidant protection by converting superoxide (O_2-) free radicals to a less aggressive molecule, H_2O_2.

Synapse: A small space between adjacent brain cells through which one cell signals another cell by transport of neurotransmitter to a receptor.

Synthesis: The production of a substance by the union of chemical elements, groups, or simpler compounds or by the degradation of a complex compound.

Synthroid (levothyroxine): A natural thyroid hormone used to treat hypothyroidism.

Tabula rasa: The theory that humans are born with a blank slate (absence of mental content) and that their personality, emotions, and knowledge result from life experiences.

Tau proteins: Proteins within brain cells that interact with tubulin to stabilize microtubules and promote tubulin assembly into microtubules. Tau protein defects have been associated with Alzheimer's disease and other forms of dementia.

Transgenerational epigenetic inheritance (TEI): A process in which altered gene expression in a person can be transferred to future generations.

Tinnitus: A false perception of sound commonly referred to as ringing in the ears that occurs without the presence of external noise.

Transaminase: An enzyme that transfers an amino group from one molecule to another.

Transdermal: A type of medication that is placed on the skin to deliver a specific dose of medication through the skin and into the bloodstream.

Transmembrane protein: A protein (often linear or globular in structure) that spans the entire cell membrane and acts as a conduit for nutrients, neurotransmitters, or other substances to enter or leave the cell.

Transporter protein (transporter): A transmembrane protein that helps a certain substance or class of closely related substances to cross the membrane. In neurotransmission, this is a membrane-spanning protein that enables rapid reuptake of a neurotransmitter from the synapse.

Treatment naïve: An adjective describing an individual who has not previously been treated for a particular condition.

Trepanation: A medical intervention in which a hole is drilled or otherwise produced in a human skull, which was an early "treatment" for mental illness aimed at the release of evil spirits.

Tricyclic amines: Antidepressant medications such as Norpramin, Amitryptyline, Elavil, etc. that have three rings of atoms in their basic chemical structure. These medications were widely used prior to the introduction of SSRI and SNRI antidepressants.

Tryptophan: An essential amino acid needed for synthesis of serotonin, growth in infancy, and nitrogen balance in adults.

Ubiquitin: A small protein comprised of 76 amino acids that is present in all human cells and has a multitude of functions including the tagging of unwanted proteins and labeling them for destruction.

Ventral tegmental area: A brain area rich in dopamine cells that has a role in pleasure, motivation, cognition, drug addiction, and emotional responses, such as fear.

Vesicle: A small pouch in the body that contains a fluid. In the brain, tiny vesicles absorb neurotransmitters for subsequent release into the synapse following cell firing.

Vesicular monoamine transporter (VMAT): A transport protein embedded in the membrane of a vesicle that facilitates loading of neurotransmitter molecules into the vesicle.

Vitamin: Any of various fat-soluble or water-soluble organic substances essential in minute amounts for normal growth and activity of the body and obtained naturally from plant and animal foods.

Wilson's disease: A rare inherited disorder of copper metabolism, characterized by excessive deposition of copper in the liver, brain, and other tissues along with depressed blood copper levels.

Zinc fingers: Small metalloproteins in which zinc is coordinated with histadine and cysteine, which have a role in genetic transcription, typically acting as interaction modules that bind to DNA, RNA, or chromatin proteins.

APPENDIX A—METHYLATION

Introduction

Methane is the simplest organic chemical, consisting of one carbon atom and four hydrogen atoms (CH_4). In biochemistry, there are hundreds of cellular processes that involve methylation, a chemical reaction in which a methyl group is attached to an atom or molecule. A methyl group (CH_3) is a methane molecule with one hydrogen atom missing. With the assistance of an enzyme, a methyl group can replace a hydrogen atom of another molecule. There are four primary types of methylation reactions that are essential to life.

- *Methylation of atoms:* An important chemical reaction in humans is methylation of metals. For example, methylation of mercury or other toxic metals impacts the availability of the toxin to the brain and other organs and influences the rate of excretion from the body.

- *Methylation of molecules:* There are hundreds of important biochemical reactions in which a methyl group is donated to a molecule. In most cases, the reaction requires a methyltransferase enzyme. Methylation of amino acids is an important mechanism for producing a wide variety of proteins in the body.

- *DNA methylation:* Gene expression (protein production) within cells is regulated by methylation at certain locations along the DNA double helix molecule. This reaction primarily occurs at regions of DNA called CpG sites where a cytosine nucleotide occurs next to a guanine nucleotide connected only by a phosphorous atom. With few exceptions, CpG methylation inhibits gene expression. The relative degree of CpG methylation can determine the rate of protein synthesis in individual cells and tissues.

- *Methylation of histone proteins:* Another process for regulating gene expression involves methylation of histones, the tiny protein aggregates that serve as structural supports for fragile DNA strands in the nucleus of every cell. These reactions usually occur at lysine or arginine sites along the linear histone proteins, resulting in compaction of the DNA, thereby restricting the access of transcription factor molecules necessary for gene expression. However, there are exceptions to this rule, and in some cases, methylation at certain histone sites can promote gene expression.

The One-Carbon Cycle

A versatile methyl donor is SAMe, a molecule found in each of the trillions of cells in the human body. SAMe is produced from methionine, an amino acid present in dietary protein. A stable SAMe concentration is essential to normal embryonic development and a multitude of chemical processes throughout life. An important means for regulating SAMe levels is the one-carbon cycle, also known as the SAM cycle or the methylation cycle. This process consists of a series of chemical reactions that produce, consume, and regenerate SAMe. A schematic diagram of the one-carbon cycle is presented in Figure A-1. This biochemical cycle consists of four primary steps:

Figure A-1. Methylation Cycle

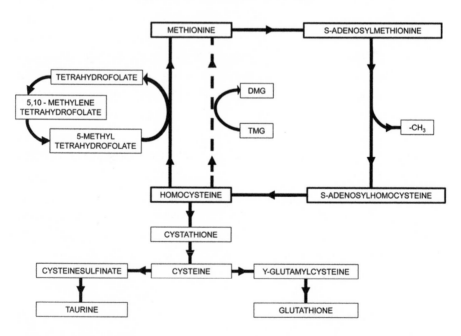

Step 1: Dietary methionine combines with adenosine triphosphate (ATP) to form SAMe. ATP is a high-energy molecule that drives the reaction with the assistance of magnesium. SAMe is a molecule that readily gives up its methyl group.

Step 2: After giving its methyl group away, SAMe is transformed into SAH (S-adenosylhomocysteine), a molecule that can be recycled to form methionine. However, if SAH builds up to excessive levels, methylation by SAMe slows down. Therefore, it is necessary for SAH to be efficiently removed by chemical reaction to enable proper methylation capability. The gold standard test for methylation status is the ratio of SAMe to SAH.

Step 3: In healthy persons, SAH is efficiently converted to homocysteine (Hcy) and proper methylation levels are maintained. The reaction involves removal of the adenosine group, assisted by an enzyme. Adenosine, in turn, is removed from the scene by adenosine deaminase (ADA), a zinc-containing enzyme. There is considerable evidence that the ADA enzyme reaction is abnormally weak in autism and other disorders.

Step 4: Part of the homocysteine is recycled to methionine, with the remainder converted to cystathionine. Both of these pathways are essential to good health: (a) recycling to methionine assists in maintenance of SAMe levels, and (b) the cystathionine pathway is a primary source of cysteine, glutathione, and other valuable antioxidants. The fraction of Hcy converted to methionine (or alternatively to cystathionine) depends on the level of oxidative stress present. It's interesting to note that high oxidative stress can cause undermethylation and also that undermethylation can cause excessive oxidative stress. The presence of either imbalance can cause the other. Recycling of Hcy to methionine can be achieved by reactions with 5-methyltetrahydrofolate (5-MeTHF) and vitamin B-12. The 5-MeTHF supplies a methyl group to form methyl-B-12, which then reacts with Hcy to produce recycled methionine. This reaction is enabled by the methionine synthase enzyme. Hcy can also convert to methionine by direct reaction with trimethylglycine (TMG), a molecule that transfers a methyl group to Hcy to form methionine and dimethylglycine (DMG).

APPENDIX B—OXIDATIVE STRESS

Oxidation is a chemical reaction that removes electrons from an atom or molecule. The term originally was used to describe reactions involving oxygen, but it has become a general term for chemical processes in which electrons are lost. In chemical reactions involving electron transfer, a reactant that donates an electron is oxidized and the reactant accepting the electron is reduced. An oxidizing agent may be thought of as a thief that attempts to steal electrons from other chemicals. There are hundreds of oxidation-reduction (redox) reactions in the human body that are essential to good health. However, many disease conditions involve oxidative stress, a condition in which natural antioxidant protectors are insufficient to prevent excessive release of free radicals and undesirable chemical reactions. Free radicals are highly reactive, unstable atoms or molecules capable of damaging proteins, membranes, DNA, and other essential biochemicals.

Modest levels of oxidative stress are needed for several essential chemical processes, including immune function. For example, oxidative stress combats bacterial infections by surrounding bacteria with H_2O_2 (a powerful oxidizing agent) that kills the unwanted organisms. In another example, superoxide and nitric oxide are oxidizing agents that regulate important processes, such as controlling vascular tone. Regulation of free radicals is accomplished by numerous antioxidant chemicals, such as glutathione, cysteine, zinc, selenium, catalase, metallothionein, and vitamins C and E. These natural biochemicals are essential to cope with environmental toxins, disease processes, and other sources of free radicals. This may be thought of as a war between the oxidative free radicals and the body's antioxidant protectors. Disease conditions can result from either overwhelming assaults by oxidative agents or insufficient levels of natural antioxidants. Conditions associated with oxidative stress include aging, heart disease, cancer, autism, Alzheimer's, and most mental illnesses. Environmental sources of oxidative stress include toxic metals, smog, pesticides, cigarettes, nuclear radiation, and industrial waste products.

Most free radicals encountered in the body can be neutralized by glutathione, zinc, catalase, melatonin, vitamin C, etc. However, the highly aggressive superoxide free radical (O_2^-) requires a special deactivation mechanism. Superoxide radicals leak from the mitochondria of all cells during natural processes and must be destroyed to avoid damage to DNA, proteins, membranes, etc. This is accomplished by a one-two punch in which a chemical known as a dismutase converts superoxide to H_2O_2 and O_2 that can be neutralized by glutathione and other antioxidants. The primary dismutases are metalloenzymes containing copper, zinc, or manganese. Ceruloplasmin, the major copper-carrying protein in the blood, also functions as a dismutase.

There has been a recent surge in research studying the role of oxidative stress in mental disorders. An increasing number of experts have proposed that oxidative stress is the primary cause of schizophrenia, bipolar disorder, autism, Alzheimer's disease, and Parkinson's disease. Advanced antioxidant therapies hold great promise for patients challenged by these disorders.

APPENDIX C—METALLOTHIONEIN

Introduction

Metallothionein (MT) proteins play an important role in mental health. Poor MT function has been associated with ADHD, autism, schizophrenia, Alzheimer's disease, and Parkinson's disease. MT proteins perform a myriad of vital functions including the following processes:

- Early brain cell development
- Powerful antioxidant capability
- Detoxification of mercury and other toxic metals
- Reduction of inflammation after injury or illness
- Enhanced efficiency of the intestinal and blood-brain barriers
- Development and functioning of the immune system
- Delivery of zinc to cells throughout the body
- Homeostatic control of zinc and copper levels in blood
- Prevention of yeast overgrowth in the intestines
- Regulation of stomach acid pH
- Taste discrimination by the tongue
- Protection of enzymes that break down casein and gluten
- Zinc signaling in brain cells
- Regulation of tumor suppression genes
- Transcription factor regulation

The Metallothionein Family of Proteins

Metallothioneins are short, linear, cysteine-rich proteins composed of between 61 and 68 amino acids. All human MTs contain 20 cysteines and have an "S" configuration with extraordinary metal binding capability. There are four varieties of metallothionein proteins. MT-I and MT-II are found throughout the body, and their functions include regulation of zinc and copper levels, development of neurons and synaptic connections, enhancement of immune function, and protection against toxic metals. MT-III is a necessary factor in the pruning and growth-inhibitory phases of brain cell development. MT-IV regulates stomach acid pH and enables taste discrimination by the tongue.

Synthesis of MT proteins involves genetic expression of thionein (induction) followed by loading of thionein with metal atoms. MT-I and MT-II take on seven zinc atoms, while MT-III typically contains four copper atoms and 3 zinc atoms. MT proteins are generated in response to injury, illness, emotional stress, or exposure to toxic metals. They represent a major antioxidant system in the body.

MT proteins are found at high levels in four brain areas: hippocampus, amygdala, pineal gland, and cerebellum. The hippocampus is essential to cognition, speech, learning, memory, and behavioral control. The amygdala has a role in emotional memory and socialization. The pineal gland produces melatonin that assists sleep. The cerebellum enables smooth physical movements. Weakened MT function could result in problems in any of these areas.

Brain Development

In infancy, the brain has a high population of small, densely packed neurons. MT-III plays an important role in pruning of brain neurons during early development, which enables the remaining brain cells to grow and develop synaptic connections. In addition, MT-III is the primary inhibitory factor that stops the growth process when brain cells reach optimal size. An early MT-III dysfunction would be expected to result in the following:

♦ Incomplete pruning
♦ Areas of densely packed undeveloped neurons
♦ Increased brain volume and head diameter

All of these phenomena have been reported in autism spectrum disorders. This understanding has led to MT-Promotion therapies aimed at completion of brain development in children. These therapies are also under development for Alzheimer's disease since extremely low MT levels have been observed in this disorder.

Detoxification of Heavy Metals

Metallothioneins are heavy metal magnets. They bind mercury, lead, cadmium, and other toxic metals tightly and render them relatively harmless. Deficiencies in metallothionein functioning would, therefore, be expected to lead to an increased burden of these dangerous substances. MT proteins work in tandem with GSH and selenium. Metal atoms are transferred into thionein by reduced GSH to form Zn_7MT. However, glutathione disulfide (GSSG) enables the release of zinc in exchange for another atom, for example, mercury, cadmium, lead, or copper. The cellular redox state of GSH determines the direction of zinc transfer. For example, GSH efficiently binds to toxic mercury but has a limited capacity. When more than 10% of reduced GSH has been converted to GSSG (oxidized GSH), the GSSG activates MT to enable its participation in sequestering toxic metals. In essence, GSH is the first defense against mercury and other heavy metals, and MT joins the fray after GSH levels have been significantly depleted. Selenium increases the kinetics of mercury transfer into MT by about 50%. Optimal protection against toxic metals requires proper amounts of GSH, MT, and selenium, and I refer to them as The Three Musketeers.

Intestinal and Blood-Brain Barriers

MT-I and MT-II are present in very high concentrations in intestinal mucosa, forming a barrier to penetration of mercury, lead, and other toxins into the portal blood stream. With respect to toxic metals, the expression leaky gut often means a failure of MT to function normally. In healthy persons, toxic metals in the diet are sequestered in mucosal MT, which is sloughed off every 5 to 10 days to be left harmlessly in the stool. It is impossible to avoid significant exposures to toxic metals in normal living, and the MT system is needed every day. For example, the average amount of mercury in a typical adult diet is about 20 micrograms/day, with higher amounts for high seafood diets. The average amount of mercury entering the body from breathing (in the USA) is one microgram/day.

MT proteins are in high concentration at the blood-brain barrier (BBB) and represent the primary protection against toxic metals from entering the brain. In addition, MT proteins within the brain assist in sequestering any toxins that penetrate the BBB. It has been estimated that in healthy adults, 90% of mercury in the diet is prevented from entering the portal blood stream that flows to the liver. In the liver, MT, GSH, and other antioxidants bind to about 90% of the mercury that has penetrated the intestinal barrier. The MT in the BBB is believed to be about 90% efficient in stopping mercury's access to the brain. In summary, less than one ingested mercury atom (or compound) in 1,000 is able to enter the brain of healthy persons. However, if MT function is weak or disabled, toxic metals can wreak havoc in the brain by altering neurotransmitter synthesis, destroying myelin, producing inflammation, increasing oxidative stress, and, in some cases, killing brain cells. Two studies have indicated MT levels are less than one-third of the normal concentration in Alzheimer's patients, and this may be a factor in the relentless death of brain cells in this disease.

Metallothionein and the GI Tract

The highest concentrations of MT proteins in the body are in the GI tract. An important role of MT in the intestines is the donation of zinc for synthesis of the enzymes carboxypepidase A and aminopepidase, which are needed to break down casein, gluten, and other proteins from food. Zinc is also required for proper functioning of dipeptidyl peptidase-IV, which breaks down gliadin, casomorphins, and other proline-containing proteins. A significant impairment in MT function could cause incomplete breakdown of casein, gluten, casomorphins, etc., which could result in severe food allergies. In my experience, about 85% of the autism population reports major lessening of symptoms after a gluten-free/casein-free diet.

MT has other important roles in the GI tract. For example, MT is an important defense mechanism against intestinal inflammation and diarrhea. In addition, MT proteins kill *Candida* and tend to prevent yeast overgrowth. Stomach parietal cells are rich in MT-IV proteins that promote formation of hydrochloric acid (HCl). MT-IV on the surface of the tongue enables taste discrimination.

Metallothionein and Immune Function

The importance of metallothionein in immune function has been known for more than 20 years. MT proteins are the primary vehicle for delivery of zinc to cells, and zinc deficiency can severely impair the immune system. In animal studies, reduced levels of MT and zinc during gestation resulted in atrophy of thymic and lymphoid tissues and greatly weakened immune response to infections. Experiments involving knockout mice (a strain of rodents with one or more genes removed—in this case an MT gene) showed severely impaired immunity.

Weak MT activity can result in a premature transition from cell-mediated immunity to humoral response and can result in a decreased amount of circulating T cells. MT also enhances immune function through its role as an efficient scavenger of free radicals. When the body is under attack by bacteria or viruses, macrophages and neutrophils work overtime to destroy the invaders. Once they have engulfed and killed an intruder, excess hydrogen peroxide is left behind, and MT is effective in mopping up this toxic oxidizing chemical.

APPENDIX D—CLINICAL RESOURCES

Physicians

There is an abundance of physicians throughout the USA and the world who provide effective therapies for ASD patients. These physicians can be found as speakers at conferences such as AutismOne (**www.autismone.org**), the National Autism Association (**www.nationalautism.org**), the Medical Academy of Pediatric Special Needs (**www.medmaps.org**), and the Autism Research Institute (**www.autism.com**). Unfortunately, there are a limited number of physicians experienced in the diagnosis and treatment of methylation imbalances, metal metabolism disorders, heavy metal overload, pyrrole disorders, fatty acid deficiency, malabsorption, glucose disorders, and other biochemical conditions that adversely impact brain function. A partial listing of doctors and clinics that provide this type of biochemical/nutrient therapy is provided below.

USA

Mensah Medical
(Dr. Albert Mensah and Dr. Judith Bowman)
4355 Weaver Parkway, Suite 110, Warrenville, IL 60555
Phone: (630) 256-8308
www.mensahmedical.com

Wyngate Health
970 Raymond Ave., Suite 101, St. Paul MN 55114
Phone: (651) 493-4566; Fax: (651) 344-0429
www.wyndgatehealth.com

Dr. Jeanne Drisko, Riordan Endowed Professor of Orthomolecular Medicine
Director, KU Integrative Medicine
University of Kansas Medical Center, Kansas City, KS 66160
Phone: (913) 588-6208
jdrisko@kumc.edu

Dr. Mary Megson (specialty—autism)
Pediatric and Adolescent Ability Center
7229 Forest Avenue, Suite 211, Richmond, VA 23226
Phone: (804) 673-9128; info@megson.com

Dr. Elizbeth Mumper (specialty—autism)
The Rimland Center for Integrative Medicine
Specialty—autism spectrum disorders
2919 Confederate Ave, Lynchburg, VA 24501
Phone: (434) 528-9075
www.rimlandcenter.com

Australia

Dr. Sharon Chant
Cooroora Family Health
5/3 Station Street, Pomona, Queensland
Phone: 07 5485 1321; Fax: 07 5335 1281

Dr. Jocelyn Cullingford
142 Cambridge St, West Leederville, Perth, Western Australia
Phone 08 9383 9997; drjcullingford@gmail.com

Dr. Marilyn Dyson, Pathways for Potential
Level 1, 4 William Street, Turramurra, New South Wales 2074
Phone: 02 9114 6800; Fax: 02 8068 2574
drdyson@pathwaysforpotential.com.au

Dr. Greg Emerson, Treat the Cause Clinic
3/400 Gregory Terrace, Spring Hill, Queensland
Phone: 07 3339 7910
www.drgregemerson.com

Dr. Kelly Francis
The Medical Sanctuary
Benowa, QLD 4217
Phone: 07 5564 5013

Dr. Frank R Golik, W.I.N. Health Coach Clinics
702 Sandgate Road, Clayfield, Queensland 4011
Phone: 07 3262 5227; Fax 07 3256 0322
recptwin@bigpond.net.au

Dr. Joanna Hickey, Wellness Medicine
41 Queens Parade, Clifton Hill, Victoria 3068
Phone: 03 9489 7955
www.wellnessmedicine.com.au

Dr. Karel Hromek
1 Argyle St, Mullumbimby, New South Wales 2482
Phone: 02 6684 3531

Dr. Carole Hungerford
Uclinic Level 1 / 421 Bourke Street, Surry Hills, New South Wales 2010
Phone: 02 9332 0400; Fax: 02 9332 2144
surryhills@uclinic.com.au

Dr. David Jaa
RPPR Services
Suite 6/140 Robina Town Centre Dr, Robina, Queensland 4226
Phone: 07 5562 2088; Fax: 07 5562 2085
www.drjaasmedicalhealth.com; www.rppr.com.au

Dr. Elizabeth Lewis
105 Lucan Street, Bendigo, Victoria 3550
Phone: 03 5441 4495; Fax: 03 5442 5558

Dr. Stephen Lyon; Woonona Medical Practice
44 Hopetoun Street, Woonona, New South Wales 2517
Phone: 02 42833433; Fax: 02 42831955
slyon@woononamedical.com.au

Dr. Shirley Mcilvenny, Natural Vibrant Health
328 Scottsdale Drive, Robina, Queensland 4226
Phone: 07 5562 5333

Dr. Nikola Ognyenovits
Brisbane, Australia
nikola@catalyst-healing.com

Dr. David Richards
Iluka Wellness Centre
51A Charles St., Iluka, New South Wales 2466
Phone: 02 6646 5082; Fax: 02 66465086

Dr. Mark Robertson
Camden Nutritional & Wellbeing Centre
44 Elizabeth St, Camden NSW 2570
Phone: 02 4655 6999

Dr. Anabel Stuckey
Suite 6, 17-19 Knox Street, Double Bay, New South Wales 2025
Phone: 02 9328 4922; Fax: 02 9328 4922
drstuckey@bigpond.com

Dr. Richard Stuckey
PO Box 484, Coolangatta, QLD 4225
Phone: 61 7 5536 4396; Fax: 61 7 5536 4045
richardstuckey@bigpond.com; www.drstuckey.com.au

Dr. Lyn Tendek
Bondi Junction Medical Practice
Level 6, Westfield Shopping Centre
500 Oxford St, Bondi Junction, New South Wales 2022
Phone: 02 9389 9699
doctorlyntendek@doctorlyntendek.com.au

Dr. Kathleen Wilson
Riverlands Therapy
PO Box 989, Penrith, New South Wales 2750
7/156 Great Western Highway, Blaxland NSW 2774
Phone: 02 47318111/ 02 47394434
Practice restricted to patients under age 25.

Dr. Mike Woodbridge
Nutritional and Environmental Medicine Queensland
Suite 7/ 20 Florence St, Teneriffe, Brisbane, Queensland 4005
Phone: 07 3831 5111
www.drmikewoodbridge.com

Ireland

Dr. Edmond O'Flaherty and Dr Andrew O'Flaherty
Gleneagle Clinic, Greygates, Blackrock, Co Dublin, Ireland
Phone: 353 12881425
eoflaherty@gmail.com

New Zealand

Dr. Kate Armstrong
Colville Community Health Centre
2299 Colville Rd, RD4, Coromandel, 3506
Phone: 07 866 6618; Fax: 07-866 6619

Norway

Hans Dahlseng
Clinical Psychologist
Funksjonellmedisinsk Senter, Huidtfeldtsgate 9a, 0253 Oslo
Phone: +47 97992500
hans@funksjonellmedisin.no; www.funksjonellmedisin.no

Dr. Eli Mohn Hove
Forusakutten A/S
Luramyrveien 79; 4013 SANDNES
Phone: 51 70 94 94

Dr. Anna Kathrine Ljøgodt
Balderklinikken
Munchsgate 7, 0165 Oslo
annakathrineljogodt@balderklinikken.no

Drs. Anne Christine Bjornebye and Sigurd Nes
Eikeliklinikken
Wilh. Wilhelmsens vei 47, 1362 Hosle
Phone: 47 67 15 93
Sig.nes@online.no

Dr. Lege Marit Rakstang
Spesialist i psykiatriFjordklinikken
Postboks 74, N-6670 Øydegard
Phone: 71 53 32 76
www.fjordklinikken.no

Philippines

Dr. Paulita Baclig
1A Paciano Rizal St., Barangay Masagana Project 4 QC
Phone: +632-5087917; Mobile: 09177065365
salutareclinica@gmail.com

Singapore

Dr Melanie Phuah
Nutramed Clinic
1 Grange Road; #10-10 Orchard Building; S239693 Singapore
Phone: +65 67350706; Fax: +65 67359589
info@nutramed.com.sg; www.nutramed.com.sg

Chemistry Laboratories
The ability to obtain accurate blood and urine levels of key biochemicals is essential
to correct diagnosis of chemical imbalances. The testing labs listed below have
demonstrated the capability for reliable measurement of these chemical factors.

Direct Healthcare Access II Laboratory
350 W. Kensington Road Suite 118
Mount Prospect, IL 60056, USA
Phone: (847) 222-9546; Fax: (847) 222-9547
info@pyroluriatesting.com

Bio-Center Laboratory
3100 North Hillside Avenue, Wichita, KS 67219 USA
Phone: (316) 682-3100; Fax: (316) 682-2062

Vitamin Diagnostics, Inc.
540 Bordertown Avenue, Suite 2300, South Amboy, NJ 08879 USA
Phone: (732) 721-1234; Fax: (732) 825-3200

Doctor's Data, Inc.
3755 Illinois Avenue; St. Charles, IL 60174-2420, U.S.A
Phone: (800) 323-2784 (USA & Canada); 0871-218-0052 (United Kingdom);
Fax: (630) 587-7860
Inquiries@doctorsdata.com

Sullivan-Nicoladies Pathology
Cnr Whitmore St & Seven Oaks St.
Taringa, Queensland 4068, Australia
Phone: 07 3377 8666; 1 800 777 877

Bio Medisinsk Laboratorium AS
Besøksadresse: Rådmann Halmrastsvei 4, 2 etg; 1337 Sandvika, Norway
Postadresse: Postboks 81, 1300 Sandvika, Norway
Phone: (+47)21063550; Fax: (+47)21063555
www.bmlab.no

Compounding Pharmacies

Compounding of prescribed nutrients can be effective in (a) improving treatment compliance and (b) providing an alternative for children and others who do not swallow capsules. Effective nutrient therapy sometimes involves a large number of individual vitamins, minerals, and amino acids, and many patients have difficulty taking numerous capsules and tablets. Compounding of the prescribed nutrients can usually reduce the number of capsules by 50-80% and ease compliance problems. In addition, small children and some adults may be unable to swallow capsules or tablets, so they require treatment using powders that can be mixed with liquids. For these patients, compounding pharmacies can pack the carefully blended nutrient ingredients into capsules. The powders can be removed from the capsules and stirred into a liquid to enable compliance.

The following is a partial list of compounding pharmacies that perform this service using high-purity nutrients.

Village Green Apothecary
5415 W. Cedar Lane, Bethesda, MD 20814
Phone: (610) 453-9079; Fax (301) 963-2702
www.myvillagegreen.com

PURE Compounding Pharmacy (specializing in autism formulations)
603 East Diehl Rd, Suite 131
Naperville, IL 60563
Phone: (630) 995-4300; Fax: (630) 995-4301
www.purecompounding.com

Tugan Compounding Pharmacy
457 Golden Four Drive
Tugun QLD 4224, Australia
Phone: 07 5534 2327

ABOUT THE AUTHOR

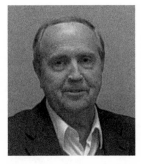

Dr. William J. Walsh is an internationally recognized expert in the field of nutritional medicine. He is president of the nonprofit Walsh Research Institute in Illinois and directs physician training programs in Australia, Norway, and other countries. Dr. Walsh has authored more than 200 scientific articles and reports and has five patents. He has presented his experimental research at the American Psychiatric Association, the US Senate, and the National Institutes of Mental Health, and he has been a speaker at 28 international conferences.

After earning degrees from Notre Dame and the University of Michigan, Dr. Walsh received a PhD in chemical engineering from Iowa State. While working at Argonne National Laboratory in the 1970s, he organized a prison volunteer program that led to studies researching the causes of violent behavior. Over the next 30 years, Dr. Walsh developed biochemical treatments for patients with behavioral disorders, ADHD, autism, depression, anxiety disorders, schizophrenia, and Alzheimer's disease that are used by doctors throughout the world.